Lippincott's Need-to-know Psychotropic Drug Facts

Katharine P. Bailey, RN, MS, CS

Assistant Professor of Nursing
Yale School of Nursing
New Haven, Connecticut

Consultant
Amy M. Karch, RN, MS

Director of Applied Science/Lecturer
Nazareth College
Rochester, New York

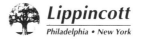

Lippincott
Philadelphia • New York

To the memory of Robert Sovner, M.D., mentor and friend

Acquisitions Editor: Margaret Zuccarini
Developmental Editor: Sara Lauber
Production Editor: Virginia Barishek
Production Manager: Helen Ewan
Production Service: Berliner, Inc.
Printer/Binder: R. R. Donnelley & Sons / Crawfordsville
Cover Designer: Jerry Cable
Cover Printer: Lehigh Press

9 8 7 6 5 4 3 2 1

Library of Congress Cataloging in Publication data

Bailey, Katharine
    Lippincott's need-to-know psychotropic drug facts / Katharine Bailey: consultant, Amy M. Karch.
      p.   cm. — (Lippincott's need-to-know)
    Includes bibliographical references and index.
    ISBN 0-7817-1039-1
    1. Psychotropic drugs—Handbooks, manuals, etc. 2. Psychiatric nursing—Handbooks, manuals, etc. I. Karch, Amy Morrison, 1949– . II. Title. III. Title: Psychotropic drug facts. IV. Series.
    [DNLM: 1. Psychotropic Drugs—nurses' instruction—handbooks. 2. Mental Disorders—drug therapy—nurses' instruction—handbooks.
QV 39 B154L 1998]
RM315.B25   1998
615'.788—DC21
DNLM/DLC
for Library of Congress
                                              97-42713
                                            CIP

Preface

This clinically focused concise pocket "quick-reference" provides "need-to-know" information on all aspects of psychotropic drugs and drugs frequently used to manage their side effects. This two-part resource provides a text overview of the pharmacologic issues concerning drug-related assessment, intervention, evaluation and patient education for drugs used to manage the common DSM-IV disorders. It includes more than 60 alphabetically organized monographs of drugs frequently administered by psychiatric nurses and nurses caring for patients with DSM-IV disorders.

The content follows the American Nurses Association (ANA) Standards of Psychiatric–Mental Health Clinical Practice Guidelines and the ANA's Psychopharmacology Guidelines for Psychiatric Mental Health Nurses (1994). A significant level of the nurse's responsibility in caring for the patient with a DSM-IV disorder is related in some way to a regimen of psychotherapeutic agents prescribed for the patient. This responsibility involves managing side effects, assessing for tolerance/dependence, identification of target symptoms, medication interactions and long-term monitoring of the patient. This quick reference is designed to provide quick access, need-to-know information to assist the nurse in carrying out this responsibility.

Organization

Lippincott's Need-to-know Psychotropic Drug Facts is organized in two parts:
- Part One: Assessment and Treatment Issues presents an overview, in text form, of important considerations influencing the effectiveness and compliance for various classes of psychotropic drugs used in treating depressive, bipolar, anxiety, eating, sleep, and psychotic disorders, and schizophrenia. This information is consistently presented using a standard format: introduction, indications, assessment, mechanisms of action, initiation of treatment (including choice of agent, management of side effects, drug–drug interaction), maintenance, and discontinuation.
- Part Two: This completely separate section presents more than

60 drug monographs in alphabetical order by generic drug name to enable quick access to important drug information.

Features

- Quick-reference format provides easy access to wanted information
- Overview of nursing psychopharmacology in one small volume presents a unique compilation of need-to-know information on the most frequently occurring DSM-IV disorders and the drugs used to manage them.
- Over 60 psychotropic drug monographs offer the most current resource of its kind available
- Complete drug monographs include Canadian drug names, detailed age-related dosing information, labeled and unlabeled uses, availability and blood level ranges not available in other drug guides
- Small trim size offers portability of a wealth of information that can be carried easily between hospital, clinic, and home-care setting
- Small price makes it easy to purchase one or many copies

Katherine P. Bailey, RN, MS, CS

Acknowledgments

We would like to thank the many people who have helped to make this book possible both directly and indirectly: our editor at Lippincott–Raven Publishers, Margaret Zuccarini, who kept the project going with great persistence and perseverance; Sara Lauber, who attended to all the minute details with unwavering cheerfulness and care; all the behind-the-scenes staff at Lippincott–Raven who contributed to the production of the book; and to all our teachers, supervisors, colleagues, and students who in one way or another enriched our knowledge and skill in the practice of psychopharmacotherapy.

Contents

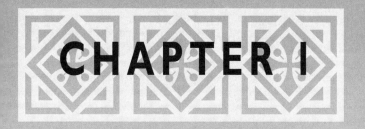

CHAPTER 1

Principles of Nursing Practice Pertaining to Psycho-pharmacologic Management

Florence Nightingale (1859) defined nursing as being in "charge of the personal health of somebody. . . [to] put the patient in the best condition for nature to act upon him." The American Nursing Association's (ANA) current definition of nursing maintains this historical perspective but also reflects nursing's evolution: Nursing is the diagnosis and treatment of human responses to actual or potential health problems.

The specialty of psychiatric–mental health nursing, as defined by the ANA in *A Statement on Psychiatric–Mental Health Clinical Nursing Practice* (1994), is the diagnosis and treatment of human responses to actual or potential mental health problems and the delivery of primary mental health care, defined as the continuous and comprehensive services necessary for:

   promotion of optimal mental health
   the prevention of mental illness
   health maintenance
   management of mental and physical health problems
   the diagnosis and treatment of mental disorders and their seque-
       lae
   rehabilitation

The scope of psychiatric–mental health nursing practice has expanded significantly as nurses within the specialty continue to assume increasing responsibility for prevention, intervention, and rehabilitation. One important aspect of psychiatric–mental health nursing care is the detection and treatment of the somatic aspects of patients' mental health problems, including indications for and responses to pharmacologic agents, usually in collaboration with other health care providers. Health teaching, including educating patients about their disorders and their medications, is an essential part of the nurse's role. Making pertinent clinical observations and judgments concerning both the therapeutic and adverse effects of prescribed drugs is of equal importance. The nursing process when applied to psychopharmacotherapy is described in the ANA's *Psychiatric–Mental Health Nursing Psychopharmacology Project* (1994) and involves: assessment, diagnosis, treatment initiation, stabilization, maintenance, and discontinuation or follow-up. A discussion of these six aspects of nursing practice as they relate to psychopharmacotherapy follows.

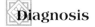

Biologic Assessment

Comprehensive and ongoing patient assessment promotes diagnostic accuracy, sound clinical judgments, and appropriate interventions. Ongoing assessment provides data used by the nurse to make modifications to the treatment plan and adjustments in psychopharmacologic management. To gather data that reflects the complete picture, the nurse should involve the patient, significant others, and interdisciplinary team members in the assessment process. Once gathered, data are synthesized, prioritized, and then documented in the medical record. The nurse should determine the priority of data collection by the client's immediate condition or need. The data may include but are not limited to:

- Baseline target symptom assessment, including the use of standardized rating scales
- Drug history, including concomitant drug use; drug allergies; and assessment of concurrent substance use, including alcohol, illicit drugs, nicotine, over-the-counter medications, and caffeine
- Assessment of appropriate patient variables, such as demographic, physical, socioeconomic, past experiences, and patient and family preferences and beliefs
- Physical, laboratory, mental status, and diagnostic assessments
- Assessment of client's ability to remain safe and not be a danger to self or others
- History of health patterns, illness, and response to prior medication

Diagnosis

Derive the diagnoses and potential problem statements from assessment data. Identify interpersonal or environmental circumstances and risk factors that may influence psychopharmacologic management. These circumstances and factors include:

- The maintenance of optimal health and well-being and the prevention of psychobiologic illness

- Deficits in the functioning of significant biological, emotional, interpersonal, and cognitive systems
- Emotional stress or crisis components of illness, pain, and disability
- Physical symptoms that occur along with altered psychological functioning
- Alterations in thinking, perceiving, symbolizing, communicating, and decision-making
- Symptom management, side effects/toxicities associated with psychopharmacologic intervention and other aspects of the treatment regimen

Use diagnostic judgments as the basis for setting treatment priorities and for selecting and assessing nursing interventions in the management of psychopharmacologic agents. Communicate these to other members of the health care team and document them in the medical record on an ongoing basis. Base diagnoses on standardized diagnostic systems such as the North American Nursing Diagnostic Association (NANDA) or other nursing system. Base psychiatric diagnoses on the *Diagnostic and Statistical Manual* (DSM)-IV.

Treatment Initiation

The primary objective of the psychiatric mental health nurse in initiating treatment is to integrate prescribed psychopharmacologic interventions into a cohesive, multidimensional plan of care to achieve optimal therapeutic response. There are many aspects to integrate when planning treatment initiation, including:

Implications of information obtained in assessment
Development of treatment plans
Informed consent
Pharmacokinetics/pharmacodynamics of prescribed agents
Patient education about medication and alternative treatments
Alternative or concurrent treatment modalities

For each patient, integrate information obtained during the nursing assessment to: [1] develop a medication treatment plan that considers target symptoms, side effects, concurrent treatments and health status, management issues regarding specific drugs, dietary and activity considerations, and patient-related variables; [2] apply knowledge regarding principles of safe and effective psychopharmacologic management, such as how dosing and tapering schedules are adjusted, indications for lab work and other prescreening or monitoring tests, and monitoring of vital signs; [3] utilize principles of health education and nursing ethics and legal parameters to inform patients about medication treatments, risk/benefits, concurrent and alternative treatments, and informed consent; [4] observe for early signs of unexpected or adverse events and initiate nursing interventions to reduce side effects and facilitate therapeutic response; [5] use the "least restrictive principle" to avoid the overuse or under use of medications as chemical restraints; [6] be cognizant of safety needs, such as potential for harm to self or others, suicidality, aggression, assaultiveness, and violence.

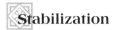

Stabilization

The stabilization phase of psychopharmacological treatment is the period of time between the first dose or initiation of treatment and the achievement of desired pharmacologic effect. Nursing objectives during this phase include implementing interventions to support the patient in achieving optimal effect. Interventions are focused on:

Continued assessment of target symptoms
Continued observation of medication effects
Continued recognition and treatment of adverse effects
Therapeutic drug monitoring by blood levels, other laboratory tests when appropriate, standardized rating scales, and patient and family reports
Alteration of medication regimens when indicated
Ongoing patient education

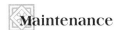

Maintenance

The maintenance phase begins when the therapeutic effect is achieved. The outcome of patient care during this period is to maintain the desired therapeutic effect for the patient. Nursing interventions during this phase of treatment include:

Ongoing monitoring of efficacy, side effects, and laboratory values
Consideration of long-term side effect potential
Addressing compliance issues
Patient education regarding relapse, relapse prevention, recognition of stressors
Consideration of possible prophylactic treatment versus discontinuation of medication treatment

To maximize the highest level of therapeutic effect, it is important to develop a psychiatric nursing plan of care in collaboration with the patient, family, and other care providers, as appropriate, based on the above objectives. Health promotion and patient education are two important areas of nursing focus. Health promotion interventions can be individualized for the patient and integrated with medication treatments, such as diet, exercise, leisure activities, and community, social, and religious affiliations. Patient education teaching includes initiating programs for relapse prevention, self-monitoring techniques and using tools such as medication cards, handouts, diaries, bibliographies, and other materials. All of these activities can be designed to encourage ongoing education of patients, families, and significant others.

Prophylaxis vs. Discontinuation and Follow-Up

The psychopharmacologic maintenance phase may be of short or long duration. During this phase, the possibility exists that the patient may need to continue on a regimen for prophylaxis or have psychopharmacotherapy discontinued. Factors to consider before making this decision include:

Recommended guidelines for the duration of treatment for any given disorder
Tapering methods/schedules
Symptom recognition
Relapse prevention

If discontinuation of a medication is recommended, include these points in the plan of care for the patient: [1] discuss the issues related to discontinuation of medication with the patient; these issues include risk/benefit considerations and potential sequelae such as withdrawal, dependence, rebound effects, and the return of symptoms of the illness; [2] develop a plan of care with the patient, family, and significant others for self-care in a postmedication phase that considers quality of life, predisposing stressors, reemergence of symptoms, appropriate use of support systems, and contact sources for potential reevaluation of treatment status; [3] carefully assess the patient just prior to tapering or discontinuing a medication and then closely monitor signs and symptoms over time after the course of treatment, clearly differentiating between changes in the patient as a result of illness effects, drug withdrawal effects, premorbid characteristics, effects of aging, and effects of the environment.

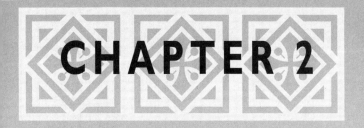

CHAPTER 2

Antidepressant Drugs

Indications for Antidepressant Agents

Antidepressant drugs are a heterogeneous group of compounds with major therapeutic effects in common. They are effective in the treatment of major depressive disorder. Some of the older antidepressants, such as the monoamine oxidase inhibitors (MAOIs), have serious side effects and are being used less often in favor of newer agents such as the serotonin-specific reuptake inhibitors (SSRIs). The SSRIs also have use in treating eating disorders and obsessive–compulsive disorders. The following are currently available categories of antidepressant agents:

Tertiary Amine Tricyclics (TCAs)	Secondary Amine Tricyclics	Tetracyclic Agents
imipramine	desipramine	maprotiline
amitriptyline	nortriptyline	amoxapine
trimipramine	protriptyline	
doxepin		
clomipramine		

Monoamine Oxidase Inhibitors (MAOIs)	Selective Serotonin Reuptake Inhibitors (SSRIs)
phenelzine	fluoxetine
tranylcypromine	sertraline
selegiline	paroxetine
	fluvoxamine

Other Compounds

    trazodone
    nefazodone
    bupropion
    venlafaxine
    mirtazepine

Antidepressant agents are effective in the treatment of a variety of other conditions including:

Prophylaxis against recurrence of major depression
Atypical depression
Panic disorder
Depression with psychotic features
Eating disorders
Body dysmorphic disorder
Chronic pain syndromes
Enuresis
Obsessive–compulsive disorder
Atypical depression

Antidepressant agents may be used with some degree of effectiveness in treating these conditions:

Attention-deficit/hyperactivity disorder
Organic mood disorders
Posttraumatic stress disorder
Social phobia

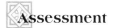 # Assessment

The best predictor of antidepressant response to drug therapy is in patients meeting the DSM-IV criteria for Major Depressive Disorder (MDD), regardless of the presence or absence of stressful life events. However, ongoing research indicates that different diagnoses may predict differential treatment response to different classes of antidepressants. Therefore, detailed assessment of target symptoms is of vital importance to accurate diagnosis and to ruling out comorbid conditions—medical as well as psychiatric. Many patients will have comorbid Axis I or II disorders with MDD.

The psychiatric conditions most often mistaken for major depressive disorders are:

dysthymic disorder
personality disorders
schizoaffective disorder
anxiety disorders
somatoform disorders

normal bereavement and grief
adjustment disorder with
    depressed mood
depression secondary to
    schizophrenia

"Secondary depression" caused by organic etiologies also may be mistaken for major depressive disorder. These organic etiologies include:

Hypoxia and other cardiovascular disorders
Neoplasms, especially of the pancreas, brain, or lung
Dysfunction of the thyroid, parathyroid, or adrenal glands
Electrolyte imbalance or uremia
Vitamin deficiencies
Immune and collagen-vascular disorders
Neurologic disorders: stroke, subdural hematoma, multiple sclerosis, Parkinson's disease, Huntington's disease, uncontrolled epilepsy, syphilis, dementia, closed head injury

Depressive symptoms also can be produced as a side effect of pharmacologic intervention resulting in misdiagnosis of MDD. Several classes of drugs may produce depressive symptoms as a side effect including antihypertensive drugs, steroids, and some drugs of abuse.

Antihypertensive Drugs	Steroids
reserpine	estrogens
beta-blockers	prednisone
alpha-methyldopa	progesterone
levodopa	corticosteroids

Drugs of Abuse	Other Drugs
alcohol	cholinergics
sedative-hypnotics	benzodiazepines
cocaine	ranitidine
other psychostimulant withdrawal	calcium channel blockers

Therapeutic Mechanisms of Actions: Antidepressants

While the precise mechanisms by which antidepressant drugs exert their therapeutic effects remain unclear, much is known about their acute actions within the nervous system. Their major interaction is with the monoamine neurotransmitter systems in the brain, including norepinephrine (NE), serotonin (5HT), and dopamine (DA).

NE and 5HT are released throughout the brain by neurons originating in the locus ceruleus and brain stem raphe nuclei. Both of these neurotransmitters interact with multiple receptors to regulate arousal, vigilance, attention, mood states, sensory processing, appetite, and other global functions. The neurotransmitters are stored in vesicles in the presynaptic neuron, migrate to the cell membrane, and are then released into the synapse via electrochemical impulses. They travel across the synaptic space and bind to specific receptor sites on the postsynaptic neuron. This action sets off a cascade of postsynaptic events associated with various brain functions.

Hypotheses of the etiology of depression involve a relative deficiency of these neurotransmitters. Three of the proposed mechanisms by which neurotransmitters may be depleted are:

1. Norepinephrine, serotonin, and dopamine can be removed from the synaptic space by reuptake into the presynaptic neuron where they are either stored again in vesicles or broken down by the enzyme monoamine oxidase.
2. Increased rates of electrochemical firing at the presynaptic membrane speed up the turnover of neurotransmitters resulting in depletion.
3. Postsynaptic receptors either increase in number or become more "sensitive," resulting in depletion.

All available antidepressants target one or more of these actions. The tricyclics, venlafaxine, and mirtazepine may block the reuptake of norepinephrine (NE) and serotonin (5HT) in varying ratios, increasing available amounts of these neurotransmitters and potentiating their actions. MAOIs target two monoamine oxidase subtypes, A and B, by inhibiting the enzymes' catabolizing action, increasing available amounts of 5HT, NE, and DA, and potentiating their actions. The SSRIs block the presynaptic reuptake of 5HT but have no significant effects on NE. Bupropion may block the presynaptic reuptake of NE and/or decrease the presynaptic firing rate, decreasing the turnover of NE and potentiating its action. Nefazodone may block, or "downregulate" postsynaptic 5HT receptor sites as well as inhibit presynaptic 5HT reuptake.

Initiation of Antidepressant Treatment

Choice of Agent

The most important considerations in choosing among these agents are efficacy and side effects. All antidepressant agents appear to be of approximately equal efficacy in the treatment of major depressive disorder in double-blind, placebo-controlled studies with randomly chosen groups of patients. There do seem to be some differences in efficacy across classes of antidepressants for subtypes of depression, and individual patients may respond preferentially to a specific agent even within the same class. However, the major clinically significant differences among the antidepressants are in their side effects, and drug choice is often based on these differences.

Side Effect Patterns of Antidepressants

While the above described antidepressant mechanisms of action are associated with their therapeutic effects, these actions may be responsible for adverse effects as well. Also, antidepressant agents have other mechanisms of action that may cause other side effects via postsynaptic blockade of muscarinic (anticholinergic), histaminic, alpha- and beta-noradrenergic receptors.

Side Effects

Table 2-1 compares the sedative, anticholinergic, and hypotensive effects of antidepressants.

- All of the TCAs and MAOIs are potentially arrhythmogenic and can cause cardiotoxicity in susceptible individuals or in overdose.
- The secondary amine TCAs, except for protriptyline, have less anticholinergic, sedative, and cardiovascular side effects than the tertiary TCAs.
- The selective serotonin reuptake inhibitors (SSRIs), bupropion, venlafaxine, trazodone, nefazodone, and mirtazepine have relatively fewer anticholinergic side effects and less cardiotoxicity.

TABLE 2-1 Sedative, Anticholinergic, and Hypotensive Effects of Antidepressants

Class	Drug	Sedative	Anti-cholinergic	Hypo-tensive
Tertiary amine TCAs	amitriptyline	+++	+++	+++
	imipramine	++	++	+++
	doxepin	+++	+++	++
	clomipramine	+++	+++	+++
	trimipramine	+++	++	++
Secondary amine TCAs	desipramine	+	+	++
	snortriptyline	+	+	+
	protriptyline	+	+++	+
SSRIs	fluoxetine	+	+/−	+/−
	sertraline	+	+/−	+/−
	paroxetine	+	+/−	+/−
	fluvoxamine	+	+/−	+/−
MAOIs	phenelzine	+	+/−	+++
	tranylcypromine	+	+/−	+++
Others	amoxapine	+	+	++
	maprotiline	++	+	++
	venlafaxine	+	+/−	+/−
	bupropion	+	+/−	+/−
	nefazodone	++	+/−	+
	trazodone	+++	+/−	++
	mirtazepine	++	+	+

+ + + = potent effect
+ + = moderate
+ = mild
+/− = questionable or absent

- Trazodone, nefazodone, mirtazepine, and the tertiary amines (TCAs) can cause sedation.
- The SSRIs, bupropion, and venlafaxine may cause nausea, headache, agitation, insomnia, or sexual dysfunction. However, all of the new agents tend to be more tolerable than the cyclic agents.

Managing Side Effects

Anticholinergic Side Effects

Anticholinergic effects include dry mouth, constipation, and urinary retention. These may be helped by the patient increasing water intake and dietary fiber. Sugarless gum, candy, or fluoride lozenges can alleviate dry mouth. Bethanechol (Urecholine) 25–50 mg three or four times a day may reduce urinary hesitancy, may ameliorate dry mouth and constipation, and may be helpful for impotence when taken 30 minutes before sexual intercourse. Stool softeners such as Colace may be helpful. Narrow-angle glaucoma can also be aggravated by anticholinergic drugs. However, TCAs and tetracyclic antidepressants can be used in patients with glaucoma, provided that pilocarpine eye drops are administered concurrently.

Postural Hypotension

Postural hypotension may respond to a variety of interventions, including salt tablets, modest amounts of caffeine, and, in severe cases, the mineralocorticoid fludrocortisone (Florinef) in doses of about 0.4 mg/day may be helpful.

Cardiac Effects

TCAs and tetracyclics can cause changes in heart rate and in conduction. Their use in patients with preexisting conduction defects is contraindicated. In patients with a cardiac history, these drugs should be initiated at low doses, with gradual increases and careful monitoring of cardiac functions.

Central Nervous System (CNS) Effects

Sedating antidepressants may be given at bedtime, or if dosing is more than once a day, the largest share of the dosage can be given at bedtime. If, on the other hand, an antidepressant is stimulating, the dosage can be given in the earlier part of the day. It appears that all antidepressants may lower the seizure threshold. Although they can still be used in patients with epilepsy or organic brain lesions (except bupropion), the initial doses should be lower and then raised more slowly than in other patients.

Allergic Effects

Skin rashes and blood dyscrasias are rare complications of antidepressant treatment. However, a complete blood count (CBC) should be done immediately if a patient shows signs of infection. In the case of rash, the drug should be discontinued until its cause can be determined.

Other Side Effects

Unwanted weight gain or loss can be managed by diet and exercise. Nausea can usually be ameliorated by taking the medication with food in the stomach.

Dose reduction is always a reasonable first step when any side effect emerges.

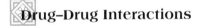

Drug–Drug Interactions

Monoamine Oxidase Inhibitors (MAOIs) and Tyramine

The most feared—although infrequent—adverse effect associated with MAOIs is the hypertensive response triggered by tyramine ingestion or the concomitant administration of certain sympathomimetic agents. Bee stings may also cause a hypertensive reaction. When patients taking MAOIs ingest food or drink that contain the amino acid tyramine, they may have a life-threatening hypertensive reaction. This is because tyramine is also broken down by the enzyme monoamine oxidase (MAO), and so inhibition of MAO in the gastrointestinal (GI) tract results in increased absorption of tyramine into the bloodstream and, potentially, a hyperadrenergic crisis with mild to severe hypertension, hyperpyrexia, tachycardia, diaphoresis, tremulousness, and cardiac arrhythmias.

Other amines besides tyramine (phenylethylamines, dopamine, and others) in foods may induce these crises in MAOI-treated patients.

Foods with a very high tyramine content (to be avoided):

Alcohol (particularly beer and wines, especially Chianti; a small
   amount of scotch, gin vodka, or sherry is permissible)
Fava or broad beans
Aged cheese (Camembert, Liederkranz, Edam, and cheddar;
   cream cheese and cottage cheeses are permitted)
Beef or chicken liver
Orange pulp
Pickled or smoked fish, poultry, or meats
Soups (packaged)
Yeast vitamin supplements
Meat extracts (e.g., Marmite, Bovril)
Summer (dry) sausage

Foods with moderately high tyramine content (no more than one or two servings a day):

Soy sauce
Sour cream
Bananas (green bananas can be included only if cooked in their
   skins; ordinary peeled bananas are fine)
Avocados
Eggplant
Plums
Raisins
Spinach
Tomatoes
Yogurt

Monoamine Oxidase Inhibitors (MAOIs) and Serotonergic Agents

Another potentially life-threatening drug interaction involves MAOIs
and agents that are serotonergic. These agents in combination with
MAOIs may result in a "serotonin syndrome," which, if mild, may fea-
ture tachycardia, hypertension, fever, ocular oscillations, muscle
rigidity, and myoclonic jerks. In its severe form, hyperthermia, coma,
convulsions, and death may occur. These drugs should be avoided
or used carefully during MAOI treatment:

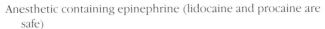

Never use:

Anesthetic containing epinephrine (lidocaine and procaine are
    safe)

Antiasthmatic medications

Antihypertensives (alpha-methyldopa, guanethidine, reserpine,
    pargyline)

Diuretics

L-Dopa, L-tryptophan

SSRIs, clomipramine

Narcotics (especially meperidine; morphine or codeine may be
    less dangerous)

Over-the-counter cold, hay fever, and sinus medications, espe-
    cially those containing dextromethorphan (aspirin, aceta-
    minophen, and menthol lozenges are safe)

Sympathomimetics (amphetamine, cocaine, methylphenidate,
    dopamine, metaraminol, epinephrine, norepinephrine, iso-
    proterenol)

Use carefully:

Antihistamines

Disulfiram

Hydralazine (Apresoline)

Propranolol (Inderal)

Terpin hydrate with codeine

Tricyclic drugs

For other drug–drug interactions between specific antidepressants and other agents, please see individual drug monographs.

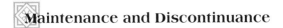

Maintenance and Discontinuance

Based on studies with TCAs, patients with unipolar depression are
at high risk for relapse if treatment is discontinued within the first 16
weeks of therapy. Therefore, in treatment responders, most experts
favor continuation for a minimum of six months to a year. Risk of
recurrence is particularly elevated in patients with a chronic course
before recovery, multiple prior episodes, or a first episode in late life.

Patients with these histories should be encouraged to continue maintenance treatment indefinitely. Full-dose therapy is required for effective prophylaxis. The most frequent reason for failure of a drug trial is inadequate dosing for an inadequate period of time. An adequate trial for antidepressants is considered to be the highest recommended dosage for at least four, but preferably six, weeks. Except for amoxapine, which possesses some neuroleptic properties and has been implicated in tardive dyskinesia, there are no known adverse effects specifically due to long-term antidepressant treatment. However, long-term experience with some of the newer compounds is limited. If a patient makes the decision to discontinue an antidepressant, risks and benefits should be discussed, the drug should be tapered under supervision rather that discontinued abruptly, and the patient should be monitored closely for symptoms of recurrence or relapse.

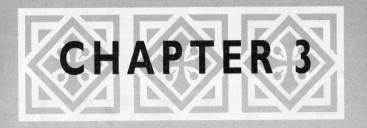

CHAPTER 3

Mood Stabilizing Drugs

All of the agents currently used as mood stabilizers to treat bipolar illness appear to be more effective in the treatment of mania than in the treatment of bipolar depression. Anticonvulsants, including valproic acid and carbamazepine, and lithium are two commonly used categories of mood stabilizing drugs. However, only two agents have labeled indications for treating mania: valproic acid and lithium.

Other drugs that have shown evidence of efficacy for the treatment of mania in either clinical trials or case reports include:

carbamazepine valproate
lamotrigine
lorazepam
nimodipine
verapamil
clonidine
diltiazem
clonazepam

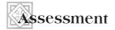Assessment

When a patient presents with depressive symptoms, the most important aspect of assessment is to differentiate bipolar from unipolar depression and/or dysphoric or mixed mania from an agitated depression. While clinical features of bipolar depression are similar to major depressive disorder (MMD), differentiating characteristics may include earlier age of onset, hypersomnia, hyperphagia, and extreme fatigue, which is sometimes referred to as "leaden paralysis."

These differentiations have important implications for pharmacologic treatment. If a patient with bipolar illness is misdiagnosed with unipolar depression and treated with an antidepressant agent, there is a risk that the antidepressant will precipitate hypomania, mania, or cause a general worsening in the patient's condition.

A hypomanic or manic episode may result from medical illness, pharmacologic treatment of a medical illness such as multiple sclerosis or hyperthyroidism, electroconvulsive therapy (ECT), or substance abuse. The following drugs can precipitate symptoms of hypomania or mania:

amphetamines
antidepressants
decongestants
corticosteroids
sympathomimetic amines

Therapeutic Mechanisms of Action of Mood Stabilizers

Lithium

Lithium has many neurobiologic effects. It is not yet certain which of these are relevant to its therapeutic mechanism of action. However, it is likely that lithium's therapeutic mechanism of action occurs when neurons are firing at high rates (as might occur in some cell groups during mania). When this happens, lithium depletes a membrane phospholipid, PIP_2, dampening the neurons' ability to respond to further stimulation by receptors that utilize this signaling pathway. Lithium may also have serotonergic properties, including sensitization of postsynaptic receptors.

Carbamazepine

Carbamazepine has two known mechanisms that may be relevant to its antiepileptic effect. It blocks, and thus inactivates, both presynaptic and postsynaptic sodium channels localized on neuronal cell bodies. The effects of these mechanisms could have widespread effects on neural function, but their relevance to mood disorders is not known.

Valproic Acid

The therapeutic mechanism of action of valproic acid is also unknown, but one possibility is that it increases levels of gamma-aminobutyric acid (GABA), the principal inhibitory neurotransmitter in the brain. The benzodiazepines, clonazepam and lorazepam, also increase levels of GABA.

Initiation of Treatment: Lithium

Indications

Lithium has been shown to be effective in bipolar disorder, both for the treatment of acute mania and for prophylaxis against recurrences. It continues to be the mainstay of the treatment of bipolar illness.

Blood Levels

Lithium therapy must be guided by measurement of serum levels. Serum level, not oral dose, is highly correlated with both therapeutic and toxic effects. Levels are usually reported as milliequivalents per liter (mEq/L). Levels are based on measurement 12 hours after the last oral dose. Serum levels will be altered by significant changes in body fluid from dehydration, polydipsia, diuretics (see below), or by salt intake, and patients should be cautioned about this. At initiation of therapy, levels should be drawn every five days (the length of time it takes for the drug to reach steady state) to adjust the dose, then every three to six months. Draw a level immediately if toxicity is suspected.

Use of lithium is complicated by its narrow therapeutic window. At serum levels only slightly higher than therapeutic, significant toxicity may occur. Even at therapeutic levels, perhaps 80% of patients experience some mild to moderate side effects. Side effects are often a particular problem at the initiation of therapy when levels are rising or when peak levels are achieved. Some patients may do better on slow-release preparations or more frequent smaller doses although this might effect compliance. Patients have varying susceptibility to toxicity which is primarily detected by clinical assessment for which serum levels provide confirmation.

The therapeutic range is usually 0.5–1.5 mEq/L. In general, some toxicity is to be expected at levels above 1.5 mEq/L; severe toxicity may manifest at levels as low as 2.0 mEq/L and is almost always evident at levels above 3.0 mEq/L.

Excretion

Lithium is excreted almost entirely by the kidney (>95%). Its excretion is not facilitated by diuretics (such as thiazides) but, in fact, reabsorption of lithium and sodium is competitive. A deficiency of sodium, as may be produced by thiazide diuretics, increases retention of lithium and, thus, increases serum lithium levels.

Lithium dosage reductions are required for patients initiating diuretic therapy, and lithium levels must be monitored closely. The diuretic furosemide blocks reabsorption of lithium to an adequate degree to not generally elevate serum lithium levels. Although lithium commonly causes defects in urine concentration ability (see below), it rarely, if ever, causes renal failure in patients whose lithium levels are maintained in the therapeutic range. Patients on long-term lithium therapy do not appear to develop significant changes in glomerular function.

Management of Side Effects

Most side effects from lithium are dose-related and most common at higher serum levels or with rapidly rising serum levels at the initiation of treatment. They are often transient, and if they occur at the initiation of treatment, the dosage can be temporarily decreased and then increased again more slowly when the symptoms abate. The first consideration in the management of side effects is to establish that the patient is on the lowest effective dose. Management of specific side effects is discussed below.

GASTROINTESTINAL EFFECTS: Nausea may be minimized if lithium is given with meals or if slow-release preparations are used, although they may result in diarrhea. Some patients may do better with lithium citrate syrup.

NEPHROGENIC DIABETES INSIPIDUS: Polyuria, polidypsia, and especially nocturia and thirst can be very troublesome to patients and may interfere with normal living habits and sleep. The diuretics furosemide or potassium-sparing amiloride may be administered because they paradoxically decrease urine output in lithium-induced polyuria. While patients on one of these diuretics can remain on a normal diet with unrestricted sodium, it is prudent to monitor weekly lithium and potassium levels for several weeks after beginning them to be sure there are no changes.

THYROID SIDE EFFECTS: Patients who develop hypothyroidism or a goiter can generally be treated by addition of thyroid hormone. It is important to perform baseline thyroid studies and follow-up studies every six months during treatment.

CARDIAC ARRHYTHMIAS: Cardiac arrhythmias are almost always reversible by discontinuation of lithium.

DERMATOLOGIC REACTIONS: Acne usually responds to vigorous treatment with standard anti-acne regimens, while psoriasis due to lithium tends to be extremely treatment resistant. When hair loss occurs, it is important to check for hypothyroidism and other possible causes of alopecia.

NEUROLOGIC SIDE EFFECTS: Lithium-associated action tremor is aggravated by anxiety and performance of fine motor movements. It may be decreased by discontinuing caffeine intake or by adding a beta-adrenergic blocker such as propranolol, starting at 10–20 mg and titrating upward as needed, or atenolol, 50 mg per day in a single daily dose. If a patient complains of severe headaches or new visual abnormalities while on lithium, a funduscopic examination should be performed to rule out lithium-associated benign intracranial hypertension.

Drug–Drug Interactions

Alcohol and other central nervous system (CNS) depressants, including prescribed psychotropic drugs and antihypertensive agents, may interact with lithium to produce sedation or confusional states. Significant drug interactions are with drugs that raise or lower blood lithium levels. These drugs include:

Drugs that raise lithium levels:
Diuretics
  thiazides
  ethacrynic acid
  spironolactone
  triamterene
Nonsteroidal anti-inflammatory agents
Antibiotics
  metronidazole
  tetracyclines
Angiotensin-converting enzyme inhibitors

Drugs that lower lithium levels:
  acetazolamide
  theophylline
  aminophylline
  caffeine (mild effect)
  osmotic diuretics

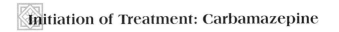

Initiation of Treatment: Carbamazepine

Indications

Carbamazepine is more effective than placebo for treatment of acute mania, but it remains uncertain whether it is as effective as lithium in long-term treatment.

Blood Levels

Therapeutic blood levels of carbamazepine in the treatment of mania appear to be in the range of 4–12 ng/ml. Carbamazepine induces its own metabolism by hepatic P450 enzymes. Therefore, a therapeutic dose that is effective early in treatment may become ineffective due to falling plasma levels after a few weeks. This autoinduction effect generally plateaus within three to five weeks. This can be confirmed by monitoring blood levels.

Management of Side Effects

Many of carbamazepine's side effects are dose related and can be decreased or eliminated by increasing the dosage slowly, by ensuring that the patient is on the lowest possible therapeutic dosage, and by giving all or most of the dosage at bedtime.

HEMATOLOGIC SIDE EFFECTS: The drug has both benign and severe hematologic toxicities. Drops in white blood cell counts are usually clinically unimportant, but rare serious or irreversible depression of red blood cells, white blood cells, or platelets have occurred. This underscores the importance of getting pretreatment CBC (complete blood count) and LFTs (liver function tests) and of monitoring these throughout the course of treatment. Patients should be instructed to report fever, sore throat, pallor, unaccustomed weakness, petechiae, easy bruising, or bleeding. Concomitant use of lithium could potentially mask carbamazepine-induced leukopenia.

Drug–Drug Interactions

Carbamazepine induces hepatic enzymes resulting in increased metabolism of itself and of certain other compounds. It has unpredictable effects on phenytoin and may augment the effects of digitalis. Other drug–drug interactions can be managed by careful dosage adjustment and careful monitoring of drug levels (see Table 3-1).

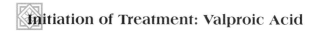

Initiation of Treatment: Valproic Acid

Indications

Valproate has been labeled for treatment of mania. It may be as effective as lithium, and some lithium-refractory patients respond to valproate alone or in combination with lithium or other antimanic drugs.

Blood Levels

There is a poor correlation between valproate serum levels and antimanic effects, but levels in the range of 50–150 ng/ml are generally required.

Management of Side Effects

Many of valproate's side effects are dose related and can be decreased or eliminated by increasing the dosage slowly, by ensuring that the patient is on the lowest possible therapeutic dosage, and by giving all or most of the dosage at bedtime.

TABLE 3-1 **Drug Interactions with Carbamazepine**

Drugs that decrease carbamazepine levels	Drugs that increase carbamazepine levels	Drug levels (effects) that are decreased by carbamazepine
phenobarbital	erythromycin	warfarin
primidone	isoniazid	ethosuximide
phenytoin	propoxyphene	valproic acid
	cimetidine	tetracycline
	SSRIs	haloperidol
		cyclic antidepressants
		benzodiazepines

Drug–Drug Interactions

See individual monograph.

General Pharmacological Management

A variety of antidepressants can be added when necessary during depressive episodes. When lithium is not effective during manic episodes or symptoms are too extreme to wait for lithium to take effect, antipsychotic agents or certain benzodiazepines can be added. For patients who do not respond to or tolerate lithium, anti-convulsants are alternatives. For rapid-cycling patients or those with mixed or dysphoric mania, anticonvulsants or clozapine may be preferable to lithium.

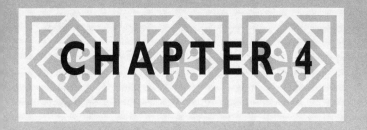

CHAPTER 4

Anxiolytic Drugs

Indications for Anxiolytics

A large variety of medications possess anxiolytic, or antianxiety, properties. Anxiolytics include the benzodiazepines and buspirone, a novel anxiolytic. There are other drugs that are also used in the treatment of anxiety even though they are not specifically labeled for this use.

Benzodiazepines

Benzodiazepines are the largest class of anxiolytic agents and are the most commonly prescribed anxiolytics in the United States. They are also classified as sedative-hypnotics. A sedative drug reduces daytime activity, tempers excitement, and is generally calming. An anxiolytic drug reduces pathological anxiety. A hypnotic drug produces drowsiness and facilitates the onset and maintenance of sleep. In general, benzodiazepines act as hypnotics in high doses, as anxiolytics in moderate doses, and as sedatives in low doses. Indications for benzodiazepines include insomnia, panic disorder, phobias, generalized anxiety disorder (GAD), alcohol withdrawal, and bipolar disorder. Zolpidem, a drug that has a similar mechanism of action as benzodiazepines but is not itself a benzodiazepine, is solely indicated for the short-term treatment of insomnia.

Currently Available Benzodiazepines

chlordiazepoxide	oxazepam	alprazolam
diazepam	lorazepam	triazolem
prazepam	temazepam	estazolam
chlorazepate	halazepam	flurazepam
midazolam	clonazepam	quazepam

Buspirone

Buspirone is a novel anxiolytic that offers a distinct alternative to benzodiazepines for the treatment of anxiety. In contrast to the benzodiazepines, buspirone carries a low potential for abuse and is not associated with withdrawal phenomena, sedation, and cognitive impairment. Its primary indication is for GAD, but it may also be effective in controlling aggression. Most available data suggest that buspirone should not be used for the treatment of panic disorder or alcohol or other sedative drug withdrawal.

Beta-Adrenergic Receptor Antagonists

Beta-adrenergic receptor antagonists, also known as beta-blockers, are used to treat the somatic symptoms of anxiety. They may reduce such symptoms as tachycardia, palpitations, tremor, and hyperventilation. Those that have been studied and used in psychiatric disorders include atenolol, metoprolol, nadolol, pindolol, and propranolol.

Some of the most effective treatments for certain anxiety disorders include serotonin reuptake inhibitors (SSRIs), tricyclics, including clomipramine, and monoamine oxidase inhibitors (MAOIs).

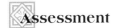 # Assessment

In assessing patients for possible anxiety disorders, there are several important considerations. First, remember that anxiety rarely occurs in isolation and is commonly accompanied by other symptoms such as depression, anger, and somatic complaints.

Another important assessment consideration is to identify or rule out anxiety secondary to medical conditions or treatments. If identified, therapy should always be directed at the underlying medical condition or to modifying the anxiety causing treatment.

As with other psychiatric disorders, the diagnosis of anxiety disorders is based on DSM-IV criteria. However, there are presentations of anxiety that are descriptively useful but do not always conform to these diagnostic categories. Descriptions of some of these follow:

Situational anxiety: reactions to a variety of stressful stimuli; usually short-lived and ends once the anticipated experience has started or when it has ended.

Phobic anxiety: a form of situational anxiety in which the primary mode of coping is avoidance.

Anticipatory anxiety: worry or apprehension preceding actual panic attacks or actual contact with dreaded objects or situations.

Traumatic anxiety: anxiety that occurs in survivors of tragic, overwhelming, usually unanticipated experiences or events.

Psychotic terror: extreme anxiety in reaction to paranoia, delusions, or hallucinations.

Anxiety associated with depression: anxiety, tension, or agitation accompanying overt depressive affect.

Stress (not an anxiety disorder nor a normative concept): anxiety precipitated by positive and negative experiences which strain or overwhelm adaptive capacities.

Anxiolytic Mechanisms of Action

The neurotransmitter gamma-aminobutyric acid (GABA) is the major inhibitory neurotransmitter in the brain. All anxiolytic benzodiazepine derivatives are active at GABA receptor sites. GABA receptors have an ion channel as well as the GABA binding site and are, therefore, referred to as the GABA-benzodiazepine receptor chloride ion channel complex.

In contrast to benzodiazepines, buspirone has no effect on GABA-receptor mechanisms but acts as an agonist on serotonin (5HT-1A) receptors. Beta-blockers modulate cardiac functions, bronchodilation, and vasodilation. Some beta-blockers (pindolol, propranolol, and nadolol) also possess serotonin (5HT-1A) antagonist activity. The anxiolytic effects of antidepressants are associated with reuptake inhibition of both serotonin and norepinephrine.

Initiation of Treatment

Choice of Drug

Because all benzodiazepines, and most likely zolpidem, have the same mechanism of action, choosing one benzodiazepine over another is based on pharmacokinetic considerations and individual patient characteristics. Dosage forms (oral, sublingual, intramuscular), rate of onset of action (rapid vs. intermediate), duration of action (1.5–160 hours), tendency to accumulate in the body, and potency vary considerably and can influence both side effects and the overall success of treatment. Table 4-1 lists clinically relevant differences between short- and long-acting agents.

There are advantages and disadvantages to both buspirone and benzodiazepines. The effects of benzodiazepines are felt within hours after they are started and the full clinical response takes only days, whereas buspirone has no immediate effect and the full clinical response may take two to four weeks. The sedative effects of benzodiazepines may be desirable, but they are also associated with impaired motor performance and cognitive deficits. Benzodiazepines have dependence and abuse potential, and withdrawal phenomena may develop upon discontinuation. Buspirone is not associated with dependence or abuse. Beta-blockers are most useful for treating the somatic symptoms of anxiety and are usually used on a p.r.n. basis, to be taken when "stage fright" or performance anxiety can be anticipated. Antidepressants are most effective for the long-term prevention of panic attacks and treatment of residual anticipatory anxiety, phobic avoidance, and obsessive-compulsive symptoms.

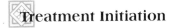

Treatment Initiation

Before starting a benzodiazepine, patients should be cautioned about possible sedation and warned not to drive or operate dangerous machinery until it is determined that their dosage does not affect performance. No specific laboratory tests are required before beginning benzodiazepines. A prior history of alcohol or other substance abuse is a relative contraindication to the use of benzodiazepines; a

TABLE 4-1 **Comparison of Long vs. Short Half-Life of Benzodiazepines**

	Long half-life	Short half-life
Advantages	• less frequent dosing • less interdose rebound anxiety or insomnia • withdrawal less problematic	• no accumulation • less next-day sedation following use for insomnia
Disadvantages	• accumulation in tissues • more risk of next-day sedation following use for insomnia	• more frequent dosing • more rebound insomnia • more interdose rebound and early morning anxiety

compelling indication, lack of an effective alternative, and careful supervision are required in this population. Other drugs used as anxiolytics (buspirone, beta-blockers, antidepressants) should be managed in the same way they are when used to treat disorders for which they have indications.

Drug–Drug Interactions

For drug–drug interactions between specific anxiolytics and other agents, see individual drug monographs and Chapter 2.

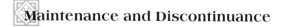

Maintenance and Discontinuance

Benzodiazepines and Tolerance, Dependence, and Withdrawal

Because of the widespread confusion of pharmacologic dependence with drug addiction and abuse, it is important for nurses to be clear about the meaning of terms that relate to dependence versus abuse:

Dependence: upon drug cessation an individual experiences significant discontinuation symptoms.

Tolerance: an individual needs a higher dosage to get the same effect.

Withdrawal: the self-limiting syndrome that includes psychological and physiologic symptoms and that occurs upon drug cessation when an individual is dependent upon the drug.

Rebound: symptoms occur soon after discontinuation and generally represent a temporary return of original symptoms but at a greater intensity than the original symptoms.

When benzodiazepines are used for short periods of time to treat anxiety states (one or two weeks in moderate doses), there is usually no evidence of tolerance, dependence, or withdrawal. The very short-acting benzodiazepines may be a slight exception to that rule, as some patients have reported increased anxiety the day after taking the drug.

The appearance of a withdrawal syndrome from benzodiazepines depends on the length of time a patient has taken the drug, the dosage the patient has been taking, the rate at which the drug is tapered, and the half-life of the particular compound. Abrupt discontinuation of benzodiazepines, particularly those with short half-lives, is associated with severe withdrawal symptoms. Serious symptoms may include paranoia, delirium, and seizures. The appearance of withdrawal symptoms may be delayed for one to two weeks in patients who had been taking benzodiazepines with very long half-lives.

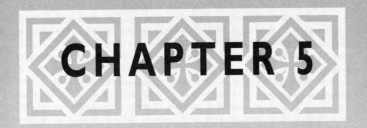

CHAPTER 5

Antipsychotic Drugs

Antipsychotic drugs have been in use for over 40 years. Because of their therapeutic mechanism of action, antipsychotic drugs are referred to as dopamine receptor antagonists. Because of their neurological and motor side effects, they also may be referred to as neuroleptics. The term "major tranquilizer" has been discarded because it mistakenly implies that the primary effect of these drugs is sedation. (See Table 5-1 for commonly used antipsychotic drugs.) The newer antipsychotic agents are referred to as serotonin and dopamine antagonists (SDAs).

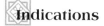 **Indications**

Antipsychotic drugs are effective in a wide variety of disorders. They have been highly effective in reducing disordered thinking, anxiety,

TABLE 5-1 Antipsychotic Drugs, Potencies, and Patterns of Side Effects

Drug	Potency	Anti-cholinergic	Extra-pyramidal	Hypo-tensive	Sedative
Chlorpromazine	low	+ + +	+ +	+ + +	+ + + +
Fluphenazine	high	+	+ + + +	+	+
Perphenazine	medium	+	+ + +	+ +	+ +
Trifluoperazine	high	+	+ + + +	+	+
Mesoridazine	low	+ +	+	+ +	+ + + +
Thioridazine	low	+ + +	+	+ + +	+ + + +
Thiothixene	high	+	+ + + +	+	+
Haloperidol	high	+/−	+ + + +	+	+
Molindone	medium	+ +	+	+/−	+
Loxapine	medium	+ +	+ + +	+ +	+ + +
Pimozide	high	+	+ + +	+/−	+
Clozapine	low	+ +	+/−	+ + +	+ + + +
Risperidone	high	+	+ +	+ +	+ + +
Olanzapine	high	+ +	+	+ + +	+ + + +

+ + + + = very significant

+ + + = significant

+ + = moderate

+ = mild

+/− = rare or absent

delusions, hallucinations, and other symptoms associated with schizophrenia. Their clinical effectiveness must be carefully evaluated, however, because of their extrapyramidal effects (EPS) and, especially, their risk of tardive dyskinesia (TD). For this reason, the long-term use of antipsychotic drugs is generally limited to the treatment of psychoses and refractory bipolar disorder. The primary indications for use of antipsychotic drugs in psychiatry include:

Schizophrenia
Acute mania and treatment-resistant bipolar illness
Depression with psychotic features
Other psychoses
Episodes of severe dyscontrol or apparent psychosis in personality disorders

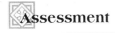

Assessment

One of the most important issues pertaining to nursing assessment of the patient receiving an antipsychotic drug is understanding the differentiating characteristics among DSM-IV psychotic disorders. These diagnoses include schizophrenia, schizophreniform disorder, schizoaffective disorder, delusional disorder, brief psychotic disorder, psychotic mania, and major depressive disorder with psychotic features. A baseline assessment of target symptoms for each patient is helpful to compare ongoing assessment findings and to evaluate the drug's therapeutic effect.

It is important to remember that substances as well as medical conditions can produce psychotic symptoms. Some examples include:

Drug-induced psychoses	Alcoholic hallucinosis
Wernicke's encephalopathy	Korsakoff's psychosis
Heavy metal intoxication	Vitamin deficiencies
Kidney and liver failure	Infections and abscesses of
Seizure disorders	the brain
Dementias	Neoplasms
Thyrotoxicosis	Lowered cardiac output
Electrolyte imbalances	Adrenal hyperfunction
CNS lupus arteritis	Diabetes mellitus

Mechanisms of Action

Therapeutic Actions of Antipsychotics

Dopamine receptor antagonism (dopaminergic blockade) is the mechanism of action thought to reduce psychotic symptoms. Most specifically, antagonism of the D2 subtype of dopamine receptor prevents the binding of dopamine (DA) to that type of dopaminergic receptor. However, because the full antipsychotic effects of these drugs may take weeks to occur, it seems likely that some long-term adaptive changes in the brain are also involved.

Some of the newer antipsychotic drugs have other therapeutic actions in addition to the D2-receptor blockade. To help distinguish the these newer agents from the older antipsychotics, the drugs have been categorized as "typical" and "atypical." The older drugs, whose primary therapeutic action is D2-receptor blockade, are referred to as "typical" antipsychotics, while the newer drugs (clozapine, risperidone, and olanzapine) are referred to as "atypical" antipsychotics. This atypical group appears to be more effective in treating negative symptoms of schizophrenia. The atypical antipsychotics block D1, D3, and D4 receptors, as well as D2 receptors, to varying degrees. And because their most potent action is the antagonism of serotonergic receptors (5HT-2), they are also referred to as serotonin–dopamine antagonists. It is this action that is thought to be responsible for their efficacy in treating the negative as well as the positive symptoms of schizophrenia.

Mechanisms of Action Associated With Side Effects

The same therapeutic actions that are responsible for the desired effects of antipsychotics, also may be responsible for some of their adverse effects. Acute dystonias, parkinsonism, akathisia, tardive dyskinesia, and endocrinological effects of antipsychotics are associated with DA blockade. Antipsychotic agents also block noradrenergic, cholinergic (muscarinic), and histaminergic receptors to varying degrees, and these actions account for a number of side effects and for some of the variation in side effect profiles among the individual drugs (see Table 5-1).

Initiation of Treatment: Antipsychotics

Choice of Agent

The efficacy of antipsychotic agents for reducing disordered think-ing, anxiety, delusions, hallucinations, and other positive symptoms associated with schizophrenia has been established by a vast num-ber of studies over the past 40 years. These studies consistently fail to substantiate differences in therapeutic effectiveness among the various antipsychotics despite many claims. The one exception to this is clozapine, which may be more effective in neuroleptic-resis-tant or neuroleptic-intolerant patients. Choice of agent is usually based on matching an individual drug's side effect profile to the indi-vidual patient's cluster of symptoms. For example, an agitated or sleepless patient might benefit from the sedating effects of chlor-promazine, while an elderly patient might not be able to tolerate the hypotensive effects of the drug. The side effect profile of any indi-vidual agent is in part determined by its potency. Low potency drugs tend to produce more sedative, antihypertensive, and anticholiner-gic side effects, while high potency agents tend to produce more EPS (see Table 5-1). In any event, the goal of treatment is to match the drug to the patient to achieve the fewest side effects at the low-est possible dose with the highest degree of clinical effectiveness.

Side Effects

Besides the side effects mentioned above, antipsychotics can pro-duce numerous other adverse effects including dermatological, oph-thalmic, cardiac, hematological, and hepatic adverse events (see individual drug monographs for specific side effects). When these side effects are life-threatening or cause intolerable discomfort to the patient, the primary interventions are either discontinuation of the offending drug or, if practical, lowering the dosage. Other strate-gies for the management of side effects resulting from antipsychotic treatment are discussed below.

Management of Side Effects

HEMATOLOGIC EFFECTS: Many blood dyscrasias may occur as a result of antipsychotic treatment, but, except for leukopenia, which is common but not serious, they are rare. Agranulocytosis, seen with all antipsychotics at an incidence of approximately 1 in 500,000, can be life-threatening. Routine complete blood counts (CBCs) are not indicated, but if a patient reports a sore throat, fever, or any other sign of infection, a CBC should be done immediately, and if the indexes are low, the drug should be stopped and the patient transferred to a medical facility. The mortality rate for this complication may be as high as 30 percent.

DYSTONIAS: About 10 percent of all patients experience dystonic reactions from antipsychotics, usually in the first few hours or days of treatment. They are most common in men less than 40 years of age but can occur at any age in either sex. They are most common with intramuscular (IM) dosages of high-potency antipsychotics. Dystonias can fluctuate spontaneously, responding to reassurance, thereby giving a false impression that the movements are hysterical and under conscious control. They are slow, contained, muscular contractions or spasms that can involve the neck, tongue, eyes, jaw, or the entire body. Some dystonias involving the mouth, tongue, jaw, neck, and pharynx can result in trouble breathing and cyanosis. Acute treatment with IM anticholinergics or related drugs or prophylaxis with oral preparations almost always relieves or prevents the symptoms.

PARKINSONIAN EFFECTS: Parkinsonian side effects occur in about 15 percent of patients treated with antipsychotics, usually within the first 3 months of treatment. Women are affected about twice as often as men, and the disorder can occur at all ages, although it is most common after age 40. High-potency neuroleptics are more likely to result in these effects. Symptoms include muscle stiffness, often referred to as "lead-pipe rigidity"; cogwheel rigidity; shuffling gait; stooped posture; coarse tremor; pill-rolling tremor; and perioral tremor, sometimes referred to as "rabbit syndrome."

These symptoms can be treated with anticholinergics, amantadine, or diphenhydramine. About 50 percent of patients need continued treatment, while the remainder develop a tolerance. After antipsychotics are withdrawn, parkinsonian symptoms may last up to three months. The anticholinergic drug should be continued in these patients until the symptoms have completely resolved.

TREMOR: Tremors associated with antipsychotics typically decrease during periods of relaxation and sleep, and increase with stress and anxiety. To minimize medication-induced tremor, patients should minimize their caffeine consumption. The drug should be taken at bedtime to minimize the amount of daytime tremor. Also, beta-blockers such as propranolol can be given to treat the tremor.

AKATHISIA: Akathisia is a subjective feeling of muscular discomfort that can cause the patient to be agitated, pace relentlessly, alternately sit and stand in rapid succession, demonstrate continuous repetitive movements such as leg swinging or rocking, and feel generally dysphoric. The symptoms cannot be controlled by the patient's will and can appear at any time during treatment. Anticholinergics or amantadine are not particularly effective for akathisia. Propranolol 30–120 mg a day, benzodiazepines, and clonidine may be more effective.

TARDIVE DYSKINESIA: Tardive dyskinesia (TD) is a delayed effect of antipsychotics; it rarely occurs until after six months of treatment. About 10–20 percent of patients who are treated with antipsychotics for more than a year develop TD. Women are more likely to be affected than men, and patients more than 50 years of age, patients with brain damage, children, and patients with mood disorders are also at high risk. Between 50 and 90 percent of all mild cases of TD remit, and between 5 and 40 percent of all cases of TD eventually remit if the drug is discontinued. This means that a significant proportion of patients who develop TD suffer from permanent symptoms. It is less likely to remit in elderly patients. The disorder consists of abnormal, involuntary, irregular choreoathetoid movements of the muscles of the head, the limbs, and the trunk. The severity of the movements ranges from minimal to grossly incapacitating. Perioral movements are the most common and include darting, twisting, and protruding movements of the tongue; chewing and lateral jaw movements; lip puckering; facial grimacing; finger movements and hand clenching. Torticollis, retrocollis, trunk twisting, and pelvic thrusting are seen in severe cases. Dyskinesia is exacerbated by stress and disappears during sleep.

TD has no single effective treatment. The basic approach is prevention and management by using antipsychotics only when clearly indicated in the lowest effective dosages. The new atypical antipsychotics may not be associated with TD, and switching to one of these is a treatment strategy. Patients who are receiving antipsychotics should be examined regularly for the appearance of abnormal movements by using the Abnormal Involuntary Movement Scale (AIMS).

NEUROLEPTIC MALIGNANT SYNDROME: Neuroleptic malignant syndrome (NMS) is a life-threatening complication that can occur anytime during the course of antipsychotic treatment. The symptoms usually evolve over 24–72 hours. The diagnosis is often missed in the early stages because the withdrawal or agitation may be mistaken for an increase in psychosis. Men are affected more commonly than women and young patients more commonly than elderly. The mortality rate can reach 20–30 percent or higher when depot antipsychotics are involved. Motor and behavioral symptoms include muscular rigidity and dystonia, akinesia, mutism, obtundation, and agitation. Autonomic symptoms include hyperpyrexia, sweating, and increased pulse and blood pressure. Laboratory findings include increased white blood cell count, creatinine phosphokinase, liver enzymes, plasma myoglobin, and myoglobinuria, occasionally associated with renal failure.

The first step in treatment is the immediate discontinuation of the drug and vigorous medical support including symptomatic treatment of fevers, close monitoring of vital signs, electrolytes, fluid balance, and renal output. Antiparkinsonian medications or the skeletal muscle relaxant dantrolene may reduce some of the muscle rigidity. The dopamine agonists amantadine or bromocriptine may decrease some of the symptoms. Treatment should be continued for 5–10 days, and when antipsychotic treatment is restarted, the patient should be switched to a different, preferably low-potency, drug.

SEDATION: The low-potency antipsychotics are the most sedating. Patients should be warned about driving or operating machinery when first treated. Giving the entire dose at bedtime may eliminate sedation problems and patients often develop tolerance to this side effect.

ORTHOSTATIC HYPOTENSION: Orthostatic hypotension occurs most frequently during the first few days of treatment, and patients readily develop a tolerance to it. It occurs most frequently when low-potency, especially IM low-potency, antipsychotics are given. The chief dangers, although uncommon, are that patients may faint or fall. Nurses should measure the patient's blood pressure (lying and standing) before and after the first dose and during the first few days of treatment. Patients should be warned and instructed to rise from bed gradually, sit with their legs dangling for a minute before getting out of bed, and sit or lie down if they feel faint. Wearing support hose may help alleviate the symptoms.

ANTICHOLINERGIC EFFECTS: Anticholinergic effects are common, especially when low-potency antipsychotics are given. The most common are dry mouth and nose, blurred vision, constipation, urinary retention, and mydriasis. Advise patients to rinse out their mouth frequently with water and to use sugarless gum or candies.

Constipation may be helped by adding fiber and water to the diet or it may be treated with the usual laxative preparations. Bethanechol 25–50 mg three or four times a day may be useful in patients with urinary retention.

ENDOCRINE EFFECTS: Antipsychotics are associated with an increased secretion of prolactin which can result in breast enlargement, galactorrhea, decreased libido, inhibited orgasm or impotence, and amenorrhea. Women may have a false pregnancy test result while taking some antipsychotics. Patients are often reluctant or embarrassed to report disturbing sexual side effects, and nurses may not find out about them unless they ask specifically. It is important that nurses ask specifically about sexual side effects throughout the course of treatment so that associated issues can be discussed with the patient and, when applicable, with the patient's sexual partner.

DERMATOLOGICAL EFFECTS: When rashes occur during antipsychotic treatment, the drug should be stopped until the cause of the rash can be determined. A variety of skin eruptions can occur early in treatment, generally in the first few weeks, and usually remit spontaneously. Patients need to be informed that this is reversible and be reassured until they do remit. A photosensitivity reaction that resembles a severe sunburn or, in some cases, a blue-gray discoloration of the skin over areas exposed to sunlight occurs in some patients. Advise patients to use sunscreen, to wear a hat and other clothing that covers the body, and to avoid the sun as much as is practically possible.

WEIGHT GAIN: This is a common side effect of antipsychotic treatment, but can be addressed by changes in diet and increased exercise. Molindone and, perhaps, loxapine are not associated with this symptom and may be indicated for patients for whom weight gain is a serious health hazard or a reason for noncompliance.

Drug–Drug Interactions

Some antipsychotic agents affect the metabolism of other drugs (e.g., tricyclic antidepressants, phenytoin), and some other drugs affect the metabolism of antipsychotics. These interactions may have important clinical consequences, most significantly, toxicity. Of particular note are the additive effects when anticholinergics are given with antipsychotics—particularly low-potency antipsychotics—to reduce EPS. In fact, incidences of toxicity are most commonly the result of drug–drug interactions. For other pharmacodynamic inter-actions between specific antipsychotics and other agents see the individual drug monographs.

Maintenance and Discontinuance

A patient with psychotic illness should continue to receive an effective dosage of an antipsychotic for at least six months after improvement. If the patient has had only one or two psychotic episodes and has been in a stable clinical state for 6 months, a very gradual dosage reduction (6–12 months) is reasonable. Patients who have had three or more exacerbations of psychotic illness should probably continue to receive antipsychotics indefinitely with possible attempts to reduce the dosage from time to time. The nurse should know enough about the patient's life to be able to identify current stressors or predict future ones so that medication can be regulated accordingly.

Because many patients treated with antipsychotic drugs have chronic or relapsing illnesses, long-term use of antipsychotics may be indicated. The nurse should discuss the risks and benefits of maintenance treatment with the patient, and should consider the patient's wishes, the severity of the illness, and the quality of the patient's support systems. Because of the risk of TD and of non-compliance due to this and other side effects, dosage should be monitored closely throughout the course of treatment, always striving for the lowest effective dosage. The prescriber should consider alternative treatments and additional supportive interventions whenever possible. When patients relapse because of noncompliance and they do not respond to psychosocial measures, consideration should be given to the use of depot preparations. Because these are long-acting preparations, patients should be exposed to the oral form of the drug prior to their first injection. It is safest to start long-acting agents at low dosages and then carefully adjust them to maximize therapeutic effect and minimize side effects.

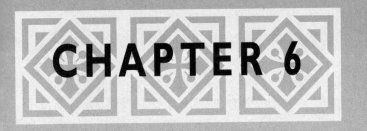

CHAPTER 6

Drug Monographs

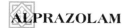ALPRAZOLAM

....

Apo-Alpraz (CAN), Novo-Alprazol (CAN), Nu-Alpraz (CAN), Xanax

PREGNANCY CATEGORY C

C-IV controlled substance

Drug Classification: *Type:* anxiolytic; *Class:* triazolo-benzodiazepine.

Mechanisms of Action
Benzodiazepines bind to specific receptor sites associated with the major inhibitory neurotransmitter in the brain, gamma-aminobutyric acid (GABA), thereby increasing the affinity of the receptor sites. While the exact mechanisms of action are not completely understood, inhibitory actions on neurons within the limbic system, and on serotonergic (5-HT) and noradrenergic neurons within the brainstem, are responsible for the anxiolytic properties.

Indications
Management of anxiety disorders and panic attacks. Premenstrual syndrome.

Depression.

Contraindications/Cautions
Contraindications: • hypersensitivity to benzodiazepines • psychoses, acute narrow-angle glaucoma, shock, coma, acute alcoholic intoxication • pregnancy (cleft lip or palate, inguinal hernia, cardiac defects, microcephaly, pyloric stenosis when used in first trimester; neonatal withdrawal syndrome reported in babies) • lactation.
   Use cautiously with: • patients with history of alcohol or drug dependence or addiction • elderly or debilitated patients • patients with impaired liver or kidney function.

Dosage
Adult: 0.5–6 mg/d; may be given bid–qid.

Pediatric Adolescent: Not for use in children <18 y.

Geriatric: Initial dose 0.25 mg/d; adjust dose according to tolerance and individual response.

Dosage Forms: Tablets: 0.25, 0.5, 1, 2 mg.

Pharmacokinetics
Absorption: from GI tract at medium rate with rapid onset of action. *Distribution:* highly lipid soluble, crosses placenta, passes into breast milk. *Metabolism:* hepatic; $T_{1/2}$: 10–15 h. *Peak plasma level:* 1–2 h. *Steady state:* up to 2 wk. *Elimination:* urine.

Adverse Effects
CNS: Transient, mild drowsi-

ness initially; sedation, fatigue, ataxia; confusion, depression, lethargy, stupor, apathy, lightheadedness, disorientation, dysarthria, headache, slurred speech, tremor, vertigo, diplopia, nystagmus, paradoxical excitatory reactions, anxiety, hallucinations, euphoria, difficulty in concentration, vivid dreams, psychomotor retardation increased muscle spasticity, insomnia, rage, sleep disturbances, minor changes in EEG patterns.

GI: Constipation, changes in salivation, nausea, anorexia, vomiting, difficulty in swallowing, elevations of blood enzymes—LDH, alkaline phosphatase, SGOT, SGPT; hepatic dysfunction, jaundice.

CV: Bradycardia, tachycardia, hypertension and hypotension, palpitations, edema.

HEMATOLOGIC: Neutropenia, blood dyscrasias.

GU: Incontinence, urinary retention, changes in libido.

DERMATOLOGIC: Skin rashes.

TOLERANCE/DEPENDENCE: Some patients report a tolerance to the anxiolytic effects of benzodiazepines and require increased doses to maintain clinical remission. There is also a cross-tolerance among most of the benzodiazepines. Abrupt discontinuation, particularly of those with short half-lives, is associated with severe withdrawal symptoms seen only in patients who have taken high doses for long periods. Appearance of the syndrome may be delayed for 1–2 wk with benzodiazepines with very long half-lives. Commonly observed withdrawal symptoms in benzodiazepine withdrawal syndrome: anxiety, irritability, insomnia, fatigue, headache, muscle twitching or aching, tremor, shakiness, sweating, dizziness, concentration difficulties, nausea, anorexia, observable depression, depersonalization, derealization, increased sensory perception, abnormal perception or sensation of movement.

Clinically Important Drug–Drug Interactions

∄ Decreased absorption with antacids.

∄ Increased CNS depression with antihistamines, barbiturates and similarly acting drugs, cyclic antidepressants, alcohol, omeprazole.

∄ Increased benzodiazepine level with cimetidine, disulfiram, erythromycin, estrogens, fluoxetine, isoniazid.

∄ Decreased benzodiazepine levels with carbamazepine and, possibly, other anticonvulsants, theophyllines, ranitidine.

Nursing Considerations

Assessment
• Assess for any of the conditions listed under "Contraindications/Cautions" above.
• Assess for current use or history of alcohol or drug dependence or abuse, use of concurrent prescribed or OTC medications.
• Patient should have had routine complete physical within last year.
• Monitor vital signs during acute alcohol withdrawal; liver and kidney function; CBC with differential during long-term therapy.
• If discontinuing, taper dosage gradually (25% per week) and monitor for withdrawal symptoms.

Drug-Specific Patient Education
• Review symptoms specific to individual patient which drug potentially treats (anxiety, panic symptoms).
• Review dosing schedule until patient demonstrates a clear understanding of regimen.
• Discuss expected onset of action.
• Review most common side effects (drowsiness, fatigue, ataxia) and encourage patient to report any side effects promptly.
• Caution patient about possible tolerance and/or psychological and physical dependence.
• Warn against abrupt discontinuation.
• Review possible withdrawal symptoms (see above under "Tolerance/Dependence").

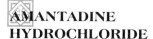

AMANTADINE HYDROCHLORIDE

••••••••••••••••••••••••••

Symadine, Symmetrel

PREGNANCY CATEGORY C

Drug Classification: *Type:* antiparkinsonian; antiviral drug; *Class:* dopamine releaser.

Mechanisms of Action
May increase dopamine release in the nigrostriatal pathway of Parkinsonism patients relieving their symptoms. Inhibits penetration of influenza virus A into the host cell.

Indications
Parkinson's disease and drug-induced extrapyramidal reactions.

Contraindications/Cautions
Contraindications: • allergy to amantadine.
   Use cautiously with:
• seizures • liver disease
• eczematoid rash • psychoses
• CHF • renal disease • lactation.

Dosage
Parkinsonism
Adult: 100 mg bid (up to 400 mg/d) when used alone; reduce

dosage in patients receiving other antiparkinsonism drugs.

Geriatric: ≥65 y, with no recognized renal disease: 100 mg once daily in Parkinsonism treatment; 100 mg bid (up to 400 mg/d) when used alone; reduce dosage in patients receiving other antiparkinsonism drugs.

Patients with Renal Disease:

Creatinine clearance (ml/min)	Dosage
10–19	Alternate 200 mg/ 100 mg every 7 d
20–29	100 mg 3 times a week
30–39	200 mg 2 times a week
40–59	100 mg/d
60–79	200 mg/100 mg on alternate days
≥80	100 mg bid

Drug-Induced Extrapyramidal Reactions
Adult: 100 mg bid PO; up to 300 mg/d in divided doses has been used.

Dosage Forms: Capsules: 100 mg; Syrup: 50 mg/5 ml.

Pharmacokinetics
Absorption: readily from the GI tract with slow onset of action (36–48 h). *Distribution:* crosses placenta and enters breast milk. *Metabolism:* not metabolized; $T_{1/2}$: 15–24 h. *Elimination:* unchanged in the urine.

Adverse Effects
CNS: Lightheadedness, dizziness, insomnia, confusion, irritability, ataxia, psychosis, depression, hallucinations.

GI: Nausea, anorexia, constipation, dry mouth.

CV: CHF, orthostatic hypotension, dyspnea.

GU: Urinary retention.

Clinically Important Drug–Drug Interactions

⋕ Increased atropine-like side effects if taken with anticholinergic drugs.

⋕ Increased amantadine effects if taken with hydrochlorothiazide, triamterene.

Nursing Considerations
Assessment
• Assess for any conditions listed under "Contraindications/Cautions" above.

• Assess for history of alcohol or drug dependence or abuse, use of current prescribed or OTC medications.

• Complete physical exam: vital signs, orientation, vision, speech, reflexes, BUN, creatinine clearance.

• Arrange to taper dosage when discontinuing—Parkinsonian crisis may occur with abrupt discontinuation.

Drug-Specific Patient Education
• Review target symptoms

that the drug potentially treats: drooling, lack of coordination, shuffling, speech impairment.

• Review dosing schedule until patient demonstrates a clear understanding of regimen and importance of continual use of drug.

• Review the most common side effects: drowsiness, blurred vision; dizziness, lightheadedness; irritability or mood changes.

• Review side effects to report promptly: swelling of the fingers or ankles; shortness of breath; difficulty urinating; tremors, slurred speech, difficulty walking.

• Caution patient not to discontinue drug abruptly as serious side effects could occur.

• Caution patient to avoid the use of alcohol, sleep-inducing drugs, or OTC drugs.

AMITRIPTYLINE HYDROCHLORIDE

• •

Elavil, Endep, Enovil, Levate (CAN), Meravil (CAN), Novotriptyn (CAN)

PREGNANCY CATEGORY C

Drug Classification: *Type:* Antidepressant; *Class:* tricyclic (TCA); *Subclass:* tertiary amine.

Mechanisms of Action

Presynaptic reuptake inhibition of neurotransmitters norepinephrine and serotonin (antidepressant efficacy is thought to be mediated by these actions). Postsynaptic blockade of histaminic, muscarinic, and noradrenergic alpha-one and alpha-two receptors (some of the undesirable side effects are thought to be mediated by these actions).

Indications

Relief of symptoms of depression (endogenous depression most responsive); sedative effects may help when depression is associated with anxiety and sleep disturbance.

Unlabeled uses: control of chronic pain; prevention of onset of cluster and migraine headaches; treatment of pathologic weeping and laughing secondary to forebrain disease.

Contraindications/Cautions

Contraindications: • hypersensitivity to any tricyclic drug • concomitant therapy with an MAO inhibitor • ECT with coadministration of TCAs • recent MI • myelography within previous 24 h or scheduled within 48 h.

Use cautiously with: • preexisting CV disorders, especially cardiac conduction system disease • seizure disorders • hyperthyroidism • angle-closure glaucoma • increased intraocular pressure • urinary retention • ureteral or urethral spasm • impaired hepatic or renal function • bipolar patients shifting to hypomanic or manic phase • elective surgery • pregnancy • lactation.

Dosage

Adult: Typical starting dose 50 mg qhs. Can be administered once a day, usually at hs. Usual maintenance dose 150–300 mg/d. Earliest onset of action in 2–5 d. Consider drug trial a failure if patient has been on maximal dose for 4–6 wk without response. Limit potentially suicidal patients' access to drug.

Pediatric Adolescent: Not recommended in children <12 y.

Geriatric: Initially 10 mg/d. Adjust dose according to tolerance and blood level.

Dosage Forms: Tablets: 10, 25, 50, 75, 100, 150 mg.

Blood Levels: Draw only to assess compliance; to confirm rapid or slow metabolizers; to document adequate drug trial. Range of therapeutic level is considered to be 100–250 ng/ml (includes sum of parent compound and desmethyl metabolite, nortriptyline); levels should be drawn when any dose has reached steady state (5–7 d) and 10–14 h after last dose.

Pharmacokinetics

Absorption: from GI tract rapidly and completely. *Distribution:* highly lipophilic and largely protein bound; crosses blood–brain barrier and placenta and enters breast milk. *Metabolism:* hepatic; $T_{1/2}$: 10–50 h. *Elimination:* urine. *Steady state:* 5–7 d.

Adverse Effects

Adult Use

CNS: Sedation and anticholinergic effects—dry mouth, blurred vision, disturbance of accommodation for near vision, mydriasis, increased intraocular pressure; confusion, disturbed concentration, hallucinations, disorientation, decreased memory, feelings of unreality, delusions, anxiety, nervousness, restlessness, agitation, panic, insomnia, nightmares, hypomania, mania, exacerbation of psychosis, drowsiness, weakness, fatigue, headache, numbness, tingling, paresthesias of extremities, discoordination, motor hyperactivity, akathisia, ataxia, tremors, peripheral neuropathy, extrapyramidal symptoms, seizures, speech blockage, dysarthria, tinnitus, altered EEG.

GI: Dry mouth, constipation, paralytic ileus, nausea, vomiting, anorexia, epigastric distress, diarrhea, flatulence, dysphagia, peculiar taste, increased salivation, stomatitis, glossitis, parotid swelling, abdominal cramps, black tongue, hepatitis.

CV: Orthostatic hypotension, hypertension, syncope, tachycardia, palpitations, MI, arrhythmias, heart block, precipitation of CHF, stroke.

HEMATOLOGIC: Bone marrow depression, including agranulocytosis; eosinophilia, purpura, thrombocytopenia.

GU: Urinary retention, delayed micturition, dilation of the urinary tract, gynecomastia, testicular swelling in men; breast enlargement, menstrual irregularity, and galactorrhea in women; increased or decreased libido; impotence

HYPERSENSITIVITY: Skin rash, pruritus, vasculitis, petechiae, photosensitization, edema (generalized, facial, tongue), drug fever.

ENDOCRINE: Elevated or depressed blood sugar, elevated prolactin levels, inappropriate ADH secretion.

WITHDRAWAL: Abrupt discontinuation of prolonged therapy: nausea, headache, vertigo, nightmares, malaise.

OTHER: Nasal congestion, excessive appetite, weight gain or loss; sweating (paradoxical effect in a drug with prominent anticholinergic effects), alopecia, lacrimation, hyperthermia, flushing, chills.

Clinically Important Drug–Drug Interactions

⸪ Increased sedation with alcohol, antihistamines, antipsychotics, barbiturates, chloral hydrate, and other sedatives.

⸪ Increased hypotension with alpha-methyldopa, beta-adrenergic blockers, clonidine, diuretics, low-potency antipsychotics.

⸪ Additive cardiotoxicity with quinidine and other class II antiarrhythmics, thioridazine, mesoridazine, pimozide.

⸪ Additive anticholinergic toxicity with antihistamines, antiparkinsonians, low-potency antipsychotics, especially thioridazine, over-the-counter sleeping medications, gastrointestinal antispasmodics and antidiarrheals.

⸪ TCAs may increase the effects of warfarin and block the effects of guanethidine.

⸪ Increased sympathomimetic (especially alpha-adrenergic) effects of direct-acting sympathomimetic drugs (norepinephrine, epinephrine).

⸪ Decreased effects of indirect-acting sympathomimetic drugs (ephedrine).

⸪ Increased levels and possible delirium with disulfiram.

Note: MAOIs and TCAs have been used successfully in some patients who are resistant to therapy with single agents;

however, hyperpyretic crises, severe convulsions, hypertensive episodes, and deaths can occur when MAOIs are given with TCAs.

Nursing Considerations

Assessment

• Assess for any of the conditions listed under "Contraindications/Cautions" above.

• Assess for ETOH or drug use/abuse and for concomitant prescribed and/or OTC medications.

• Complete physical exam: vital signs, EKG for patients 40 y or older, CBC with differential, thyroid function, liver function, BUN, creatinine, weight changes, I & O, vision; sexual interest, function, and activity.

Drug-Specific Patient Education

• Review target symptoms that drug potentially treats: disruptions in sleep, appetite, concentration, energy, mood; anhedonia; interest; motivation; initiative.

• Review dosing schedule until patient demonstrates a clear understanding of regimen.

• Discuss expected lag period (3–4 wk) before therapeutic effects can be anticipated.

• Review most common side effects: dry mouth, constipation, dizziness, urinary hesitancy, headache, nausea, sedation, or agitation, and encourage patient to report any side effects promptly.

• Caution patient against abrupt discontinuation without consulting prescriber. Abrupt discontinuation may cause withdrawal symptoms (cholinergic rebound, malaise, chills, coryza, muscle aches, agitation, insomnia) or rapid reemergence of depressive symptoms.

• Caution patient about ETOH or drug use.

BENZTROPINE MESYLATE

••••••••••••••••••••••••

Apo-Benztropine (CAN), Cogentin, PMS Benztropine (CAN)

PREGNANCY CATEGORY C

Drug Classification: *Type:* antiparkinsonian; *Class:* anticholinergic.

Mechanisms of Action

Has anticholinergic activity in the CNS that is believed to help normalize the hypothesized imbalance of cholinergic/ dopaminergic neurotransmission in the basal ganglia of the brains of Parkinsonism patients. Reduces severity of rigidity, and, to a lesser extent, akinesia and tremor; less effective overall than levodopa. Peripheral anticholinergic effects suppress secondary symptoms of Parkinsonism such as drooling.

Indications

Adjunct in the therapy of Parkinsonism (postencephalitic, arteriosclerotic and idiopathic types).

Control of extrapyramidal disorders (except tardive dyskinesia) due to neuroleptic drugs (e.g., phenothiazines).

Contraindications/Cautions

Contraindications: • hypersensitivity to benztropine • glaucoma, especially angle-closure glaucoma • pyloric or duodenal obstruction, stenosing peptic ulcers, achalasia (megaesophagus) • prostatic hypertrophy or bladder neck obstructions • myasthenia gravis.

Use cautiously with: • tachycardia • cardiac arrhythmias • hypertension • hypotension • hepatic or renal dysfunction • alcoholism • chronic illness • people who work in hot environment • hot weather • lactation.

Dosage

Adult: *Parkinsonism:* Initially 0.5–1 mg PO hs; a total daily dose of 0.5–6 mg given hs or in 2–4 divided doses is usual. Increase initial dose in 0.5 mg increments at 5–6-d intervals to the smallest amount necessary for optimal relief. Maximum daily dose is 6 mg. May also be given parenterally (IM or IV) in same dosage as orally. When used concomitantly with other drugs, gradually substitute benztropine for all or part of the other medication and gradually reduce dosage of the other drug.

Drug-induced extrapyramidal symptoms: Acute dystonic reactions: Initially 1–2 mg IM (preferred) or IV to control condition. May repeat if Parkinsonian effect begins to return. After that, 1–2 mg PO bid to prevent recurrences. *Extrapyramidal disorders occurring early in neuroleptic treatment:* 1–2 mg PO bid–tid. Withdraw drug after 1–2 wk to determine its continued need; reinstitute if disorder reappears.

Pediatric Adolescent: Safety and efficacy not established.

Geriatric: Strict dosage regulation may be necessary; patients >60 often develop increased sensitivity to the CNS effects of anticholinergic drugs.

Dosage Forms: Tablets: 0.5, 1, 2 mg; Parenteral 1 mg/ml.

Blood Levels: Utility has not been established.

Pharmacokinetics

Absorption: rapid from GI tract. *Distribution:* crosses blood brain barrier, crosses placenta and enters breast milk. *Metabolism:* hepatic; peak level, 1 h. *Duration:* 6–10 h. *Elimination:* unknown.

Adverse Effects
Peripheral Anticholinergic Effects

GI: Dry mouth, constipation, dilation of the colon, paralytic ileus, nausea, vomiting, epigastric distress.

EYE: Blurred vision, mydriasis, diplopia, increased intraocular tension, angle-closure glaucoma.

CV: Tachycardia, palpitations, hypotension, orthostatic hypotension.

GU: Urinary retention, urinary hesitancy, dysuria, difficulty achieving or maintaining an erection.

SKIN: Skin rash, urticaria, other dermatoses.

OTHER: Flushing, decreased sweating, elevated temperature.

CNS Effects, Some of Which Are Characteristic of Centrally Acting Anticholinergic Drugs

CNS: Disorientation, confusion, memory loss, hallucinations, psychoses, agitation, nervousness, delusions, delirium, paranoia, euphoria, excitement, lightheadedness, dizziness, depression, drowsiness, weakness, giddiness, paresthesia, heaviness of the limbs.

OTHER: Muscular weakness, muscular cramping; inability to move certain muscle groups (high doses), numbness of fingers.

Clinically Important Drug–Drug Interactions

⊯ Paralytic ileus, sometimes fatal, when given with other anticholinergic drugs or with drugs that have anticholinergic properties (phenothiazines, tricyclic antidepressants).

⊯ Additive adverse CNS effects—toxic psychosis—with other drugs that have CNS anticholinergic properties (tricyclic antidepressants, phenothiazines).

⊯ Possible masking of the development of persistent extrapyramidal symptoms, tardive dyskinesia, in patients on long-term therapy with antipsychotic drugs (phenothiazines, haloperidol).

⊯ Decreased therapeutic efficacy of antipsychotic drugs (phenothiazines, haloperidol) possibly due to central antagonism.

Nursing Considerations
Assessment

• Assess for any of the conditions listed under "Contraindications/Cautions" above.

• Assess for ETOH and drug use/abuse and for prescription and/or OTC medications.

• Complete physical exam: vital signs, skin color, lesions, orientation, affect, reflexes, bilateral grip strength, visual exam including tonometry, liver and kidney function tests.

Drug-Specific Patient Education

• Review target symptoms that the drug potentially treats: tremor, drooling, shuffle, lack of coordination.

• Review dosage schedule until patient demonstrates a clear understanding of the regimen; emptying the bladder before each dose may be helpful.

• Review the most common side effects: drowsiness, dizziness, confusion, blurred vision; nausea; dry mouth; painful or difficult urination; constipation; weakness and fainting in hot weather.

• Review side effects to report promptly: difficult or painful urination; constipation; rapid or pounding heartbeat; confusion; eye pain or rash

• Caution patient to avoid the use of alcohol, sedative, and OTC drugs.

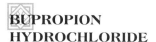

BUPROPION HYDROCHLORIDE

••••••••••••••••••••••••

Wellbutrin, Wellbutrin SR

PREGNANCY CATEGORY B

Drug Classification: *Type:* Unicyclic antidepressant; *Class:* aminoketone (structurally related to phenylethylamines, amphetamines, and diethylpropion).

Mechanisms of Action

Poorly understood. Antidepressant effect appears to be associated with inhibition of presynaptic dopamine transporter. Weak blocker of serotonin and norepinephrine. Minimal anticholinergic activity.

Indications

Treatment of depression and attention-deficit/hyperactivity disorder.

Contraindications/Cautions

Contraindications: • hypersensitivity to bupropion
• history of seizure disorder, bulimia or anorexia, head trauma, CNS tumor • pregnancy
• lactation • renal or liver disease • heart disease or history of MI.

Dosage

Adult: Begin 100 mg bid; may be increased to maximum dose as tolerated. Because of the risk of seizures (0.4%), recommended total daily dose of bupropion should be no higher than 450 mg and that no individual dose no higher than 150 mg given no more frequently than q 6 h. Slow release (SR) tablets: Begin with 150 mg q a.m., and increase to target dose of 150 mg bid. Doses should be given 8 h apart. Maximum dose: 200 mg bid. Earliest onset of action within 2–5 d. Consider drug trial a failure if patient has been on maximum recommended dose for 4–6 wk without response.

Pediatric Adolescent: Safety and efficacy in children <18 y not established.

Geriatric: Start at 50 mg q a.m., and increase as tolerated. Use with caution and monitor geriatric patients carefully.

Dosage Forms: Tablets: 75, 100 mg; Slow release (SR) tablets: 100, 150 mg.

Pharmacokinetics

Absorption: well-absorbed from the GI tract. *Distribution:* 80% protein bound; may cross placenta; may pass into breast milk. *Metabolism:* hepatic; $T_{1/2}$: 8–24 h; SR $T_{1/2}$: 20–37 h. *Steady state:* within 8 d *Elimination:* urine and feces.

Adverse Effects

CV: Palpitation, flushing, migraine, hot flashes.

GI: Dry mouth, nausea, constipation, diarrhea, anorexia, nausea, vomiting, dysphagia.

MUSCULOSKELETAL: Myalgia, arthralgia, arthritis, twitch.

CNS: Insomnia, dizziness, agitation, anxiety, tremor, nervousness, somnolence, irritability, memory decrease, paresthesia, CNS stimulation.

RESPIRATORY: Pharyngitis, sinusitis, increased cough.

SKIN: Sweating, rash, pruritus, urticaria.

SPECIAL SENSES: Tinnitus, taste perversion, amblyopia.

GU: Urinary frequency, urinary urgency, vaginal hemorrhage, urinary tract infection.

OTHER: Headache, infection, abdominal pain, asthenia, chest pain, pain, fever.

Clinically Important Drug–Drug Interactions

‡ Carbamazepine, phenobarbital, phenytoin may decrease bupropion levels.

‡ Cimetidine may increase levels of bupropion.

‡ Potential drug interactions may exist between bupropion and drugs that affect the cytochrome P4502B6 metabolism (e.g., orphenadrine and

cyclophosphamide).

- Acute toxicity of bupropion may be enhanced by phenelzine.
- Increased risk of adverse effects with levodopa.
- Increased risk of seizures with drugs that lower seizure threshold.

Nursing Considerations

Assessment

- Assess for any of the conditions listed in "Contraindications/Cautions" above.
- Assess for concurrent prescription, OTC, or illegal drug use/abuse; ETOH use/abuse; risk of suicide. Limit potentially suicidal patients' access to drug.
- Complete physical, vital signs, weight; CBC with differential; liver and thyroid function tests; BUN; creatinine; ECG if >40 y.

Drug-Specific Patient Education

- Review target symptoms that drug potentially treats: disruptions in sleep, appetite, concentration, energy, mood; anhedonia; interest; motivation; initiative; suicidal ideation.
- Review dosing schedule until patient demonstrates a clear understanding of regimen.
- Caution patient against taking more than 150 mg or 200 mg SR in one dose or more than 450 mg qd due to increased seizure risk.
- Discuss expected lag period (3–4 wk) before therapeutic effects can be anticipated.
- Review most common side effects (agitation, anxiety, dizziness, dry mouth, insomnia, nausea, sweating, anorexia, palpitation) and encourage patient to report any side effects promptly.
- Educate patient about contraception during drug use.
- Caution patient against abrupt discontinuation without consulting prescriber.
- Caution patient about concurrent ETOH and drug use.

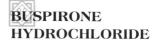

BUSPIRONE HYDROCHLORIDE

BuSpar

PREGNANCY CATEGORY B

Drug Classification: *Type:* Antianxiety agent; *Class:* azaspirodecanedione.

Mechanisms of Action

Binds serotonin receptors, has moderate affinity for dopamine receptors, and may act as a presynaptic dopamine agonist. Increases norepinephrine levels in the locus ceruleus. The clinical significance of any of these actions is not known. Lacks anticonvulsant, sedative, or muscle relaxant properties of other antianxiety agents.

Indications

Management of anxiety disorders or the short-term relief of the symptoms of anxiety.
Unlabeled use: decreasing the symptoms (aches, pains, fatigue, cramps, irritability) of premenstrual syndrome (PMS)—25 mg/d

Contraindications/Cautions

Contraindications: • hypersensitivity to buspirone • marked liver or renal impairment • lactation.
Use cautiously with: • the elderly • pregnancy.

Dosage

Adult: Initially 15 mg/d PO (5 mg tid). Increase dosage 5 mg/d at intervals of 2–3 d, as needed, to achieve optimal therapeutic response. Do not exceed 60 mg/d. Divided doses of 20–30 mg/d are commonly employed.

Pediatric Adolescent: Safety and efficacy for children <18 y not established.

Dosage Forms: Tablet: 5, 10 mg.

Blood Levels: Utility has not been established.

Pharmacokinetics

Absorption: rapid from the GI tract. *Distribution:* highly plasma protein-bound; crosses placenta and enters breast milk. *Metabolism:* hepatic; $T_{1/2}$: 3–11 h; peak level: 40–90 min. *Steady state:* 7–10 d. *Elimination:* urine.

Adverse Effects

CNS: Dizziness, headache, nervousness, insomnia, light-headedness, excitement, dream disturbances, drowsiness, decreased concentration, anger-hostility, confusion, depression, tinnitus, blurred vision, numbness, paresthesia, incoordination, tremor, depersonalization, dysphoria, noise intolerance, euphoria, akathisia, fearfulness, loss of interest, dissociative reaction, hallucinations, suicidal ideation, seizures, altered taste and smell, involuntary movements, slowed reaction time.

GI: Nausea, dry mouth, vomiting, abdominal/gastric distress, diarrhea, constipation, flatulence, anorexia, increased appetite, salivation, irritable colon and rectal bleeding.

CV: Nonspecific chest pain, tachycardia/palpitations, syncope, hypotension, hypertension.

RESPIRATORY: Hyperventilation, shortness of breath, chest congestion.

GU: Urinary frequency, urinary hesitancy, dysuria, increased or decreased libido, menstrual irregularity, spotting

OTHER: Musculoskeletal aches and pains, sweating, clamminess, sore throat, nasal congestion.

Clinically Important Drug–Drug Interactions

⚄ Increased sedation and impaired motor and mental abilities with alcohol, other CNS depressants.

⚄ Decreased effects of buspirone if taken with fluoxetine

Nursing Considerations

Assessment

• Assess for any of the conditions listed under "Contraindications/Cautions" above.

• Assess for ETOH and drug use/abuse and for prescription and/or OTC medications.

• Complete physical exam: body weight, vital signs, skin color, liver and kidney function tests, urinalysis, CBC and differential.

Drug-Specific Patient Education

• Review target symptoms that the drug potentially treats: symptoms of anxiety.

• Review dosing schedule until patient demonstrates a clear understanding of regimen.

• Review expected lag period (3–4 wk for optimum results; 7–10 d for some improvement).

• Review most the common side effects: drowsiness, dizziness, lightheadedness; GI upset; dreams, nightmares, difficulty concentrating or sleeping, confusion, excitement.

• Review side effects to report promptly: abnormal involuntary movements of facial or neck muscles, motor restlessness; sore or cramped muscles; abnormal posture; yellowing of the skin or eyes.

• Caution patient to report pregnancy immediately.

• Caution patient to avoid the use of alcohol, sleep-inducing, or OTC drugs.

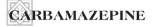

CARBAMAZEPINE

Apo-Carbamazepine (CAN), Novo-Carbamaz (CAN), Tegretol

PREGNANCY CATEGORY C

Drug Classification: *Type:* anticonvulsant; *Class:* iminostilbene (related to the TCAs).

Mechanisms of Action

Mechanism of action is not completely understood. Antiepileptic activity may be related to its ability to inhibit polysynaptic responses and block posttetanic potentiation.

Indications

Refractory seizure disorders: partial seizures with complex symptoms (psychomotor, temporal lobe epilepsy); generalized tonic-clonic (grand mal) seizures; mixed seizure patterns or other partial or generalized seizures. Carbamazepine should be reserved for patients who have not responded satisfactorily to other agents, whose seizures are difficult to control, or patients experiencing marked side effects such as excessive sedation.

Trigeminal neuralgia (tic douloureux): treatment of pain associated with true trigeminal neuralgia; also beneficial in glossopharyngeal neuralgia.

Unlabeled uses: neurogenic diabetes insipidus; certain psychiatric disorders, including bipolar disorders, schizoaffective illness, resistant schizophrenia and dyscontrol syndrome associated with limbic system dysfunction; alcohol withdrawal

Contraindications/Cautions

Contraindications: • hypersensitivity to carbamazepine or tricyclic antidepressants • history of bone marrow depression • concomitant use of monoamine oxidase inhibitors (MAOIs) • lactation.

Use cautiously with: • history of adverse hematologic reaction to any drug • glaucoma or increased intraocular pressure • history of cardiac, hepatic or renal damage • psychiatric patients (may activate latent psychosis).

Dosage

Adult: *Epilepsy:* Initial dose of 200 mg PO bid on the first day; increase gradually by up to 200 mg/d, in divided doses q 6–8 h, until the best response is obtained. Do not exceed 1200 mg/d in patients >15 y; in rare instances, doses up to 1600 mg/d have been used in adults. *Maintenance:* Adjust to minimum effective level, usually 800–1200 mg/d.

Trigeminal neuralgia: Initial dose of 100 mg PO bid on the first day; may increase by up to 200 mg/d using 100 mg increments q 12 h as needed. Do not exceed 1200 mg/d. *Maintenance:* control of pain can usually be maintained with 400–800 mg/d (range 200–1200 mg/d). Attempt to reduce the dose to the minimum effective level or to discontinue the drug at least once every 3 mo.

Combination therapy: When added to existing antiepileptic therapy, do so gradually while other antiepileptics are maintained or discontinued.

Pediatric Adolescent: *Children >12 y:* Use adult dosage. Do not exceed 1000 mg/d in patients 12–15 y, 1200 mg/d in patients >15 y.

Children 6–12 y: Initial dose is 100 mg PO bid on the first day. Increase gradually by adding 100 mg/d at 6–8 h intervals until the best response is obtained. Do not exceed 1000 mg/d. Dosage may also be calculated on the basis of 20–30 mg/kg/d, in divided doses tid–qid.

Children <6 y: Safety and efficacy not established.

Geriatric: Use caution, drug may cause confusion, agitation.

Dosage Forms: Chewable tablets: 100 mg; Tablets: 200 mg; Suspension: 100 mg/5 ml.

Blood Levels: Therapeutic levels between 4 and 12 mcg/ml.

Pharmacokinetics

Absorption: from the GI tract with slow onset of action. *Distribution:* crosses blood brain barrier; crosses placenta and enters breast milk. *Metabolism:* hepatic; $T_{1/2}$: 25–65 h, then 12–17 h. *Elimination:* urine and feces.

Adverse Effects

CNS: Dizziness, drowsiness, unsteadiness, disturbance of coordination, confusion, headache, fatigue, visual hallucinations, depression with agitation, behavioral changes in children, talkativeness, speech disturbances, abnormal involuntary movements, paralysis and other symptoms of cerebral arterial insufficiency, peripheral neuritis and paresthesias, tinnitus, hyperacusis, blurred vision, transient diplopia and oculomotor disturbances, nystagmus, scattered punctate cortical lens opacities, conjunctivitis, ophthalmoplegia, fever, chills, inappropriate antidiuretic hormone syndrome (SIADH).

GI: Nausea, vomiting, gastric distress, abdominal pain, diarrhea, constipation, anorexia, dryness of mouth or pharynx, glossitis, stomatitis. Abnormal liver function tests, cholestatic and hepatocellular jaundice, fatal hepatitis, fatal massive hepatic cellular necrosis with total loss of intact liver tissue.

HEMATOLOGIC: Potentially fatal hematologic disorders.

GU: Urinary frequency, acute urinary retention, oliguria with hypertension, renal failure, azotemia, impotence, proteinuria, glycosuria, elevated BUN, microscopic deposits in urine.

RESPIRATORY: Pulmonary hypersensitivity characterized by fever, dyspnea, pneumonitis or pneumonia.

SKIN: Pruritic and erythematous rashes, urticaria, Stevens–

Johnson syndrome, photosensitivity reactions, alterations in pigmentation, exfoliative dermatitis, alopecia, diaphoresis, erythema multiforme and nodosum, purpura, aggravation of lupus erythematosus.

CV: Congestive heart failure, aggravation of hypertension, hypotension, syncope and collapse, edema, primary thrombophlebitis, recurrence of thrombophlebitis, aggravation of coronary artery disease, arrhythmias and AV block; fatal cardiovascular complications.

Clinically Important Drug–Drug Interactions

⌘ Increased serum levels and manifestations of toxicity with erythromycin, troleandomycin, cimetidine, danazol, isoniazid, propoxyphene, verapamil—dosage of carbamazepine may need to be reduced (reductions of about 50% are recommended when given with erythromycin)

⌘ Increased CNS toxicity when given with lithium.

⌘ Increased risk of hepatotoxicity when given with isoniazid (MAOI) because of the chemical similarity of carbamazepine to the tricyclic antidepressants, and because of the serious adverse interaction documented for the TCAs and MAOIs.

⌘ Decreased absorption when given with charcoal.

⌘ Decreased serum levels and decreased effects of carbamazepine when taken with barbiturates.

⌘ Increased metabolism but no loss of seizure control when given with phenytoin, primidone.

⌘ Increased metabolism of phenytoin, valproic acid given with carbamazepine.

⌘ Decreased anticoagulant effect of warfarin, oral anticoagulants with carbamazepine.

⌘ Decreased effects of nondepolarizing muscle relaxants, haloperidol if taken concurrently.

⌘ Decreased antimicrobial effects of doxycycline given with carbamazepine.

Nursing Considerations

Assessment

• Assess for any condition listed under "Contraindications/Cautions" above.

• Assess for history of alcohol or drug dependence or abuse, use of current prescribed or OTC medications.

• Complete physical exam: vital signs, ophthalmologic exam (including tonometry, funduscopy, slit-lamp exam), CBC including platelet and reticulocyte counts, serum iron, hepatic function tests, urinalysis, BUN, thyroid function tests, EEG.

• Assure that drug is only used for indications listed; it should be reserved for use for epileptic seizures that are refractory to other safer agents.

• Arrange to reduce dosage, discontinue carbamazepine, or substitute other antiepileptic medication gradually. Abrupt discontinuation of all antiepileptic medication may precipitate status epilepticus.

• Arrange for frequent liver function tests; arrange to discontinue drug immediately if hepatic dysfunction occurs.

• Arrange for patient to have CBC, including platelet, reticulocyte counts, and serum iron determination, before initiating therapy, weekly for the first 3 mo of therapy, and monthly thereafter for at least 2–3 y. Arrange to discontinue drug if there is evidence of marrow suppression, as follows:

Erythrocytes	<4 million/mm^3
Hematocrit	<32%
Hemoglobin	<11 g/100 ml
Leukocytes	<4000/mm^3
Platelets	<100,000/mm^3
Reticulo-cytes	<0.3% (20,000/mm^3)
Serum iron	>150 mcg/100 ml

Drug-Specific Patient Education

• Review the target symptoms that the drug potentially treats: decreased number of seizures, relief of pain of trigeminal neuralgia.

• Review the dosing schedule, until patient demonstrates a clear understanding of regimen; take drug with food to decrease GI upset, do not discontinue drug abruptly.

• Review the most common side effects: drowsiness, dizziness, blurred vision; GI upset.

• Review the side effects patient should report promptly: bruising, unusual bleeding, abdominal pain, yellowing of the skin or eyes, pale-colored feces, darkened urine, impotence, CNS disturbances, edema, fever, chills, sore throat, mouth ulcers, skin rash, pregnancy.

• Caution patient about the need for frequent check-ups, including blood tests, while on this drug.

• Caution patient to use contraceptive techniques at all times.

• Caution patient not to discontinue drug abruptly.

• Caution patient to avoid the use of alcohol and sleep-inducing or OTC drugs.

CHLORDIA-ZEPOXIDE HYDROCHLORIDE

••••••••••••••••••••••••

Apo-Chlordiazepoxide (CAN), Librium, Libritabs, Mitran, Reposans-10, Solium (CAN)

PREGNANCY CATEGORY D

C-IV controlled substance

Drug Classification: *Type:* anxiolytic; *Class:* 2-keto-benzodiazepine

Mechanisms of Action

Benzodiazepines bind to specific receptor sites associated with the major inhibitory neurotransmitter in the brain, gamma-aminobutyric acid (GABA), thereby increasing the affinity of the receptor sites. While the exact mechanisms of action are not completely understood, inhibitory actions on neurons within the limbic system, and on serotonergic (5-HT) and noradrenergic neurons within the brainstem, are responsible for the anxiolytic properties.

Indications

Relief of symptoms of anxiety. Symptomatic relief of acute alcohol withdrawal.

Contraindications/Cautions

Contraindications: • hypersensitivity to benzodiazepines • psychoses • acute narrow-angle glaucoma • shock • coma • acute alcoholic intoxication • pregnancy (cleft lip or palate, inguinal hernia, cardiac defects, microcephaly, pyloric stenosis when used in first trimester; neonatal withdrawal syndrome reported in babies) • lactation.

Use cautiously with: • patients with history of alcohol or drug dependence or addiction • elderly or debilitated patients • patients with impaired liver or kidney function.

Dosage

Adult: Usual range (oral and parenteral): 15–100 mg/d; oral may be given bid–qid.

Pediatric Adolescent: >6 y: 5–30 mg/d; <6 y: not recommended.

Geriatric: Initial dose 5 mg/d; adjust dose according to tolerance and remission of symptoms.

Dosage Forms: Tablets: 5, 10, 25 mg; Capsules 5, 10, 25 mg; Parenteral 100 mg.

Pharmacokinetics

Absorption: from GI tract at medium rate with rapid onset of action. *Distribution:* highly lipid soluble, crosses placenta, passes into breast milk. *Metabolism:* hepatic; $T_{1/2}$: 24–48 h. *Peak plasma level:* (oral) 1–4 h,

(IM) 15–30 m. *Steady state:* up to 2 wk. *Elimination:* urine.

Adverse Effects

CNS: Transient, mild drowsiness initially; sedation, fatigue, ataxia; confusion, depression, lethargy, stupor, apathy, light-headedness, disorientation, dysarthria, headache, slurred speech, tremor, vertigo, diplopia, nystagmus, paradoxical excitatory reactions, anxiety, hallucinations, euphoria, difficulty in concentration, vivid dreams, psychomotor retardation increased muscle spasticity, insomnia, rage, sleep disturbances, minor changes in EEG patterns.

GI: Constipation, changes in salivation, nausea, anorexia, vomiting, difficulty in swallowing, elevations of blood enzymes—LDH, alkaline phosphatase, SGOT, SGPT; hepatic dysfunction, jaundice.

CV: Bradycardia, tachycardia, hypertension and hypotension, palpitations, edema.

HEMATOLOGIC: Neutropenia, blood dyscrasias.

GU: Incontinence, urinary retention, changes in libido.

DERMATOLOGIC: Skin rashes.

TOLERANCE/DEPENDENCE: Some patients report a tolerance to the anxiolytic effects of benzodiazepines and require increased doses to maintain clinical remission. There is also a cross-tolerance among most of the benzodiazepines. Abrupt discontinuation, particularly of those with short half-lives, is associated with severe withdrawal symptoms seen only in patients who have taken high doses for long periods. Appearance of the syndrome may be delayed for 1–2 wk with benzodiazepines with very long half-lives. Commonly observed withdrawal symptoms in benzodiazepine withdrawal syndrome: anxiety, irritability, insomnia, fatigue, headache, muscle twitching or aching, tremor, shakiness, sweating, dizziness, concentration difficulties, nausea, anorexia, observable depression, depersonalization, derealization, increased sensory perception, abnormal perception or sensation of movement.

Clinically Important Drug–Drug Interactions

‡ Decreased absorption with antacids.

‡ Increased CNS depression with antihistamines, barbiturates and similarly acting drugs, cyclic antidepressants, alcohol, omeprazole.

‡ Increased benzodiazepine level with cimetidine, disulfiram, erythromycin, estrogens, fluoxetine, isoniazid.

‡ Decreased benzodiazepine

levels with carbamazepine and, possibly, other anticonvulsants, theophyllines, ranitidine.

Nursing Considerations

Assessment
• Assess for any of the conditions listed under "Contraindications/Cautions" above.
• Assess for history of alcohol or drug dependence or abuse, use of concurrent prescribed or OTC medications.
• Patient should have had routine complete physical within last year.
• Monitor vital signs during alcohol withdrawal; liver and kidney function; CBC with differential during long-term therapy.
• If discontinuing, taper dosage gradually (25% per week) and monitor for withdrawal symptoms.

Drug-Specific Patient Education
• Review symptoms specific to individual patient which drug potentially treats (anxiety, alcohol withdrawal, panic, phobias, insomnia).
• Review dosing schedule until patient demonstrates a clear understanding of regimen.
• Discuss expected onset of action.
• Review most common side effects (drowsiness, fatigue, ataxia) and encourage patient to report any side effects promptly.

• Caution patient about possible tolerance and dependence.
• Warn against abrupt discontinuation.
• Review possible withdrawal symptoms (see above under "Tolerance/Dependence").

CHLORPROMAZINE HYDROCHLORIDE
••••••••••••••••••••••••••••

Largactil (CAN), Thorazine

PREGNANCY CATEGORY C

Drug Classification: *Type:* dopamine receptor antagonist; also called antipsychotic, neuroleptic, or major tranquilizer; *Class:* phenothiazine; *Subclass:* aliphatic.

Mechanisms of Action
Postsynaptic antagonism of dopamine receptors, primarily D2 (antipsychotic efficacy is thought to be mediated by these actions). Blockade of muscarinic cholinergic, noradrenergic, and histaminergic receptors (some undesirable side effects are thought to be mediated by these actions).

Indications
Short- and long-term management of idiopathic psychoses

including schizophrenia, schizophreniform disorder, schizoaffective disorder, delusional disorder, brief psychotic disorder, mania with psychosis, and major depressive disorder with psychotic features.

Secondary psychoses associated with a general medical condition or substance-related disorder.

Acute deliria and organic psychoses.

Severe agitation or violent behavior.

Severe behavioral problems in children marked by combativeness and/or explosive hyperexcitability and in the short-term treatment of hyperactive children who show excessive motor activity.

Movement disorder of Huntington's disease.

Motor and vocal tics of Tourette's Syndrome.

Brief use for episodes of severe dyscontrol or apparent psychosis in some personality disorders.

Control of nausea, vomiting, and intractable hiccups.

Contraindications/Cautions

Contraindications: • allergy to chlorpromazine • comatose or severely depressed states • presence of large amounts of CNS depressants (alcohol, barbiturates, narcotics, etc.) • bone marrow depression • blood dyscrasias • circulatory collapse • subcortical brain damage • Parkinson's disease • liver damage • cerebral or coronary arteriosclerosis • CV disease • severe hypotension or hypertension • respiratory disorders • glaucoma • history of epilepsy or seizures • peptic ulcer or history of peptic ulcer • decreased renal function • urinary retention, ureteral or urethral spasm • prostate hypertrophy • breast cancer • thyrotoxicosis • myelography within 24 h or scheduled within 48 h • pregnancy • lactation • exposure to heat, organophosphorous insecticides, or atropine or related drugs • children with chickenpox • CNS infections • if signs and symptoms of tardive dyskinesia appear, drug discontinuation should be considered • history of neuroleptic malignant syndrome.

Dosage

Adult: Patients may respond to widely different dosages of antipsychotics. Therefore, there is no set dosage for any given antipsychotic drug. Usual range for acute use (oral): 300–1000 mg/d. Usual range for maintenance use (oral): 100–600 mg/d. Can be administered once a day.

IM: oral forms should be used whenever possible, but IM forms may be necessary for patients who exhibit violent behavior or for those who have high first-pass or presystemic metabolism of oral forms. Starting dose 25 mg IM; may repeat in 1 h; increase dosage gradually up to 400 mg q 4–6 h. Switch to oral dosage as soon as patient is able or willing.

Pediatric Adolescent: Generally not used in children <6 mo; 0.5 mg/kg PO q 4–6 h; 1 mg/kg rectally q 6–8 h; 0.5 mg/kg IM q 6–8 h; not to exceed 40 mg/d (up to 5 y) or 75 mg/d (5–12 y).

Geriatric: Start dosage at one-fourth to one-third that given in younger adults and increase more gradually.

Dosage Forms: Tablets: 10, 25, 50, 100, 200 mg; Sustained release forms: 30, 75, 150, 200, 300 mg; Liquid concentrate: 30 mg/ml; 100 mg/ml; Syrup: 10 mg/5 ml; Injection: 25 mg/ml; 10 mg/ml.

Pharmacokinetics

Absorption: (oral) adequate but variable; food or antacids may decrease absorption; liquid preparations are absorbed more rapidly and reliably than tablets; onset of action 3–60 min; peak level: 2–4 h; IM rapidly and reliably absorbed; onset of action 15–20 min; peak: 30–60 min. *Distribution:* highly protein bound (85–90%) and lipophilic; readily crosses the blood–brain barrier, placenta, and enters breast milk; concentrations in the brain appear to be greater than those in blood; not removed efficiently by dialysis. *Metabolism:* hepatic. *Elimination:* urine. The elimination half-life of most antipsychotic drugs is 18–40 h; plasma levels may vary among individuals by 10- to 20-fold.

Adverse Effects

CNS: Drowsiness, insomnia, vertigo, headache, weakness, tremors, ataxia, slurring of speech, cerebral edema, seizures, exacerbation of psychotic symptoms, extrapyramidal syndromes (EPS), neuroleptic malignant syndrome, tardive dyskinesia, pseudo-parkinsonism, akathisia (see descriptions of symptoms under "Implementation" below).

GI: Dry mouth, salivation, nausea, vomiting, anorexia, constipation, paralytic ileus.

CV: Hypotension, orthostatic hypotension, hypertension, tachycardia, bradycardia, cardiac arrest, CHF, cardiomegaly, refractory arrhythmias, dysrhythmias, pulmonary edema.

RESPIRATORY: Bronchospasm,

laryngospasm, dyspnea, suppression of cough reflex, and potential aspiration.

HEMATOLOGIC: Eosinophilia, leukopenia, leukocytosis, anemia, aplastic anemia, hemolytic anemia, thrombocytopenic or nonthrombocytopenic purpura, pancytopenia, elevated serum cholesterol.

GU: Urinary retention, polyuria, incontinence, priapism, ejaculation inhibition, male impotence, urine discolored pink to red-brown.

EENT: Nasal congestion, glaucoma, photophobia, blurred vision, miosis, mydriasis, deposits in the cornea and lens, pigmentary retinopathy.

HYPERSENSITIVITY: Jaundice, urticaria, angioneurotic edema, laryngeal edema, photosensitivity, eczema, asthma, anaphylactoid reactions, exfoliative dermatitis, contact dermatitis.

ENDOCRINE: Lactation, breast engorgement in females, galactorrhea, syndrome of inappropriate ADH secretion, amenorrhea, menstrual irregularities, gynecomastia, changes in libido, hyperglycemia, inhibition of ovulation, infertility, pseudopregnancy, reduced urinary levels of gonadotropins, estrogens, and progestins.

OTHER: Fever, heat stroke, pallor, flushed facies, sweating.

Clinically Important Drug–Drug Interactions

⧫ Additive anticholinergic effects and possibly decreased antipsychotic efficacy with anticholinergic drugs.
⧫ Additive CNS depression and hypotension with barbiturates, alcohol, meperidine.
⧫ Additive effects of both drugs with beta-blockers.
⧫ Increased risk of tachycardia, hypotension with epinephrine, norepinephrine.
⧫ Increased risk of seizure with metrizamide.
⧫ Decreased hypotension effect with guanethidine.
⧫ Because of displacement and competition for protein-binding sites, concomitant treatment with other highly protein-bound medications (e.g., warfarin, digoxin) could alter concentrations of both drugs.
⧫ Decreased effect of oral anticoagulants.
⧫ Possible increase in phenytoin levels.

Lab Test Interference

• False-positive pregnancy tests (less likely if serum test is used).
• Increase in protein-bound iodine, not attributable to an increase in thyroxine.
• Blood levels of antipsychotics have not correlated well with clinical response and

serum levels are probably more misleading than useful.

Nursing Considerations

Assessment

• Assess for any of the conditions listed under "Contraindications/Cautions" above.

• Assess for alcohol and drug use/abuse and for concomitant use of prescription and/or OTC medications.

• Assess for risk of suicidality.

• Complete physical exam: vital signs including orthostatic BP, ECG, CBC with differential, thyroid and liver function, BUN, creatinine.

Implementation

• Bioavailability differs between brand names of oral forms or rectal suppositories.

• Dilute liquid concentrate just before administration in 60 ml or more of fruit juice, milk, simple syrup, orange syrup, carbonated beverage, coffee, tea, water, or semisolid foods.

• Protect liquid concentrate from light.

• Give IM injection slowly into upper outer-quadrant of buttock.

• Be alert to potential for aspiration because of suppressed cough reflex.

• Monitor for dehydration, renal or liver abnormalities, depressed WBC, symptoms of infection, cardiac arrhythmias. Promptly report to prescriber and institute remedial measures.

• Monitor for extrapyramidal side effects (involuntary dystonic muscular movements of the neck, jaw, tongue, or entire body; swallowing difficulties; oculogyric crisis); Parkinsonism (muscle stiffness; cogwheel rigidity; shuffling gait, stooped posture, drooling, coarse tremor, "rabbit syndrome," masklike facies, bradykinesia, akinesia); akathisia (subjective feeling of muscular discomfort that can cause agitation, restlessness, pacing, rocking, continually changing posture, and dysphoria).

• Monitor for symptoms of neuroleptic malignant syndrome: muscle rigidity; altered mental status; evidence of autonomic instability (e.g., irregular pulse or blood pressure, tachycardia, cardiac dysrhythmias); hyperpyrexia, sweating; increased WBC, blood creatinine phosphokinase, liver enzymes, myoglobin; mutism, obtundation, agitation.

• Monitor for symptoms of tardive dyskinesia (abnormal, involuntary, irregular, choreoathetoid movements of muscles of the head, limbs, and trunk; darting, twisting, and protruding movements of the tongue; chewing and lateral jaw movements; lip puckering; facial grimacing; finger movements and hand clenching; torticollis, retrocollis, trunk twisting, pelvic thrusting).

• Taper drug gradually after high-dose therapy due to possible gastritis, nausea, dizziness, headache, tachycardia, insomnia after abrupt withdrawal.

Drug-Specific Patient Education

• Review target symptoms that drug potentially treats: auditory, visual, olfactory, tactile hallucinations; delusions; paranoia; disorders of thought and speech; psychotic agitation; insomnia.

• Review dosing schedule until patient demonstrates a clear understanding of regimen. Caution patient against changing dosage or discontinuation without consulting prescriber.

• Caution patient against concurrent alcohol or drug use.

• Discuss expected lag period (6 wk or more) before full therapeutic effects appear.

• Review most common side effects (drowsiness, insomnia, dry mouth, constipation, dizziness from hypotension, urinary hesitancy or retention, photosensitivity, blurred vision, urticaria, EPS, Parkinsonism, akathisia), and encourage patient to report any side effects promptly.

• If possible, give the patient full information about the risk of tardive dyskinesia and possible irreversibility. (The decision whether to inform patients and/or their guardians must obviously take into account the clinical circumstances and the competency of the patient to understand the information provided.)

• Educate patient about possibly life threatening blood dyscrasias and instruct patient to report fever, chills, sore throat, unusual bleeding or bruising, or rash and to discontinue medication immediately (most likely between 4th and 10th weeks of treatment).

• Caution patient about risk of dehydration, heat stroke, and increased sensitivity to sunburn, and warn against over exercising in a hot climate.

CLOMIPRAMINE HYDROCHLORIDE

••••••••••••••••••••••••••

Anafranil

PREGNANCY CATEGORY C

Drug Classification: *Type:* Antidepressant; *Class:* tricyclic (TCA); *Subclass:* tertiary amine.

Mechanisms of Action

Presynaptic reuptake inhibition of neurotransmitters serotonin (primarily) and norepinephrine (antidepressant efficacy is thought to be mediated by these actions); may also effect dopaminergic neurotransmission. Postsynaptic blockade of histaminic, muscarinic, and noradrenergic alpha-one and alpha-two receptors (some of the undesirable side effects are thought to be mediated by these actions).

Indications
Treatment of obsessive-compulsive disorder (OCD); relief of symptoms of depression (endogenous depression most responsive).
Unlabeled uses: relief of symptoms of anxiety, panic, phobias, chronic pain, Tourette's Syndrome.

Contraindications/Cautions
Contraindications: • hypersensitivity to any tricyclic drug • concomitant therapy with an MAO inhibitor • ECT with coadministration of TCAs • recent MI • myelography within previous 24 h or scheduled within 48 h.
  Use cautiously with: • preexisting CV disorders, especially cardiac conduction system disease • seizure disorders • hyperthyroidism • angle-closure glaucoma • increased intraocular pressure • urinary retention • ureteral or urethral spasm • impaired hepatic or renal function • bipolar patients shifting to hypomanic or manic phase • elective surgery • pregnancy • lactation.

Dosage
Adult: Typical starting dose 25 mg qhs. Can be administered once a day, usually at hs. Usual maintenance dose 150–250 mg/d. Earliest onset of action in 2–5 d. Consider drug trial a failure if patient has been on maximal dose for 4–6 wk without response. Limit potentially suicidal patients' access to drug.

Pediatric Adolescent: Initially 25 mg/d. Adjust dosage according to tolerance and blood level.

Geriatric: Initially 25 mg/d. Adjust dose according to tolerance.

Dosage Forms: Capsules: 25, 50, 75 mg.

Blood Levels: Utility has not been established.

Pharmacokinetics
Absorption: from GI tract rapidly and completely. *Distribution:* highly lipophilic and largely protein bound; crosses blood–brain barrier and placenta and enters breast milk. *Metabolism:* hepatic; $T_{1/2}$: 20–30 h. *Elimination:* bile, feces. *Steady state:* 5–7 d.

Adverse Effects
Adult Use
  CNS: Sedation and anticholinergic effects—dry mouth, blurred vision, disturbance of accommodation for near vision,

mydriasis, increased intraocular pressure; confusion, disturbed concentration, hallucinations, disorientation, decreased memory, feelings of unreality, delusions, anxiety, nervousness, restlessness, agitation, panic, insomnia, nightmares, hypomania, mania, exacerbation of psychosis, drowsiness, weakness, fatigue, headache, numbness, tingling, paresthesias of extremities, discoordination, motor hyperactivity, akathisia, ataxia, tremors, peripheral neuropathy, extrapyramidal symptoms, seizures, speech blockage, dysarthria, tinnitus, altered EEG.

GI: Dry mouth, constipation, paralytic ileus, nausea, vomiting, anorexia, epigastric distress, diarrhea, flatulence, dysphagia, peculiar taste, increased salivation, stomatitis, glossitis, parotid swelling, abdominal cramps, black tongue, hepatitis.

CV: Orthostatic hypotension, hypertension, syncope, tachycardia, palpitations, MI, arrhythmias, heart block, precipitation of CHF, stroke.

HEMATOLOGIC: Bone marrow depression, including agranulocytosis; eosinophilia, purpura, thrombocytopenia.

GU: Urinary retention, delayed micturition, dilation of the urinary tract, gynecomastia, testicular swelling in men; breast enlargement, menstrual irregularity, and galactorrhea in women; increased or decreased libido; impotence.

HYPERSENSITIVITY: Skin rash, pruritus, vasculitis, petechiae, photosensitization, edema (generalized, facial, tongue), drug fever.

ENDOCRINE: Elevated or depressed blood sugar, elevated prolactin levels, inappropriate ADH secretion.

WITHDRAWAL: Abrupt discontinuation of prolonged therapy: nausea, headache, vertigo, nightmares, malaise.

OTHER: Nasal congestion, excessive appetite, weight gain or loss; sweating (paradoxical effect in a drug with prominent anticholinergic effects), alopecia, lacrimation, hyperthermia, flushing, chills.

Clinically Important Drug–Drug Interactions

⇍ Increased sedation with alcohol, antihistamines, antipsychotics, barbiturates, chloral hydrate, and other sedatives.
⇍ Increased hypotension with alpha-methyldopa, beta-adrenergic blockers, clonidine, diuretics, low-potency antipsychotics.
⇍ Additive cardiotoxicity with quinidine and other class II antiarrhythmics, thioridazine, mesoridazine, pimozide.

⊞ Additive anticholinergic toxicity with antihistamines, antiparkinsonians, low-potency antipsychotics, especially thioridazine, over-the-counter sleeping medications, gastrointestinal antispasmodics and antidiarrheals.

⊞ TCAs may increase the effects of warfarin and block the effects of guanethidine.

⊞ Increased sympathomimetic (especially alpha-adrenergic) effects of direct-acting sympathomimetic drugs (norepinephrine, epinephrine).

⊞ Decreased effects of indirect-acting sympathomimetic drugs (ephedrine).

⊞ Increased levels and possible delirium with disulfiram.

Note: MAOIs and TCAs have been used successfully in some patients who are resistant to therapy with single agents; however, hyperpyretic crises, severe convulsions, hypertensive episodes, and deaths can occur when MAOIs are given with TCAs.

Nursing Considerations

Assessment

• Assess for any of the conditions listed under "Contraindications/Cautions" above.

• Assess for ETOH or drug use/abuse and for concomitant prescribed and/or OTC medications.

• Complete physical exam: vital signs, EKG for patients 40 y or older, CBC with differential, thyroid function, liver function, BUN, creatinine, weight changes, I & O, vision; sexual interest, function, and activity.

Drug-Specific Patient Education

• Review target symptoms that drug potentially treats: obsessions or compulsions, disruptions in sleep, appetite, concentration, energy, mood; anhedonia; interest; motivation; initiative.

• Review dosing schedule until patient demonstrates a clear understanding of regimen.

• Discuss expected lag period (3–4 wk) before therapeutic effects can be anticipated.

• Review most common side effects: dry mouth, constipation, dizziness, urinary hesitancy, headache, nausea, sedation, or agitation, and encourage patient to report any side effects promptly.

• Caution patient against abrupt discontinuation without consulting prescriber. Abrupt discontinuation may cause withdrawal symptoms (cholinergic rebound, malaise, chills, coryza, muscle aches, agitation, insomnia) or rapid reemergence of depressive symptoms.

• Caution patient about ETOH or drug use.

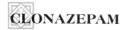CLONAZEPAM

Klonopin, Rivotril (CAN)

PREGNANCY CATEGORY D

C-IV controlled substance

Drug Classification: *Type:* antiepileptic; anxiolytic; *Class:* nitro-benzodiazepine

Mechanisms of Action

Benzodiazepines bind to specific receptor sites associated with the major inhibitory neurotransmitter in the brain, gamma-aminobutyric acid (GABA), thereby increasing the affinity of the receptor sites. While the exact mechanisms of action are not completely under-stood, inhibitory actions on neu-rons within the limbic system, and on serotonergic (5-HT) and noradrenergic neurons within the brainstem, are responsible for the anxiolytic properties.

Indications

Used alone or as adjunct in treatment of akinetic and my-oclonic seizures.

May be useful in patients with absence seizures.

Treatment of anxiety, panic, phobias, manic episodes and adjuvant to lithium therapy.

"Restless leg movements" during sleep.

Multifocal tic disorders.

Contraindications/Cautions

Contraindications: • hyper-sensitivity to benzodiazepines • psychoses, acute narrow-angle glaucoma, shock, coma, acute alcoholic intoxication • pregnancy (cleft lip or palate, inguinal hernia, cardiac defects, microcephaly, pyloric stenosis when used in first trimester; neonatal withdrawal syndrome reported in babies) • lactation.

Use cautiously with: • pa-tients with history of alcohol or drug dependence or addiction • elderly or debilitated patients • patients with impaired liver or kidney function.

Dosage

Adult: 0.5–10 mg/d; may be given in divided doses.

Pediatric Adolescent: Up to 10 y or 30 kg: 0.01–0.2 mg/kg per day; may be given qd-tid.

Geriatric: Initial dose 0.5 mg/at hs; adjust dose according to tolerance and individual re-sponse.

Dosage Forms: Tablets: 0.5, 1, 2 mg.

Pharmacokinetics

Absorption: from GI tract at rapid rate with rapid onset of action. *Distribution:* highly lipid soluble, crosses placenta, passes into breast milk. *Metab-olism:* hepatic; $T_{1/2}$: up to 50 h. *Peak plasma level:* 1–2 h.

Steady state: up to 2 wk. *Elimination:* urine.

Adverse Effects

CNS: Transient, mild drowsiness initially; sedation, fatigue, ataxia; confusion, depression, lethargy, stupor, apathy, light-headedness, disorientation, dysarthria, headache, slurred speech, tremor, vertigo, diplopia, nystagmus, paradoxical excitatory reactions, anxiety, hallucinations, euphoria, difficulty in concentration, vivid dreams, psychomotor retardation increased muscle spasticity, insomnia, rage, sleep disturbances, minor changes in EEG patterns.

GI: Constipation, changes in salivation, nausea, anorexia, vomiting, difficulty in swallowing, elevations of blood enzymes—LDH, alkaline phosphatase, SGOT, SGPT; hepatic dysfunction, jaundice.

CV: Bradycardia, tachycardia, hypertension and hypotension, palpitations, edema.

HEMATOLOGIC: Neutropenia, blood dyscrasias.

GU: Incontinence, urinary retention, changes in libido.

DERMATOLOGIC: Skin rashes.

TOLERANCE/DEPENDENCE: Some patients report a tolerance to the anxiolytic effects of benzodiazepines and require increased doses to maintain clinical remission. There is also a cross-tolerance among most of the benzodiazepines. Abrupt discontinuation, particularly of those with short half-lives, is associated with severe withdrawal symptoms seen only in patients who have taken high doses for long periods. Appearance of the syndrome may be delayed for 1–2 wk with benzodiazepines with very long half-lives. Commonly observed withdrawal symptoms in benzodiazepine withdrawal syndrome: anxiety, irritability, insomnia, fatigue, headache, muscle twitching or aching, tremor, shakiness, sweating, dizziness, concentration difficulties, nausea, anorexia, observable depression, deperson-alization, derealization, increased sensory perception, abnormal perception or sensation of movement.

Clinically Important Drug–Drug Interactions

⯾ Decreased absorption with antacids.

⯾ Increased CNS depression with antihistamines, barbiturates and similarly acting drugs, cyclic antidepressants, alcohol, omeprazole.

⯾ Increased benzodiazepine level with cimetidine, disulfiram, erythromycin, estrogens, fluoxetine, isoniazid.

⯾ Decreased benzodiazepine levels with carbamazepine and,

possibly, other anticonvulsants, theophyllines, ranitidine.

Nursing Considerations

Assessment
• Assess for any of the conditions listed under "Contraindications/Cautions" above.
• Assess for current use or history of alcohol or drug dependence or abuse, use of concurrent prescribed or OTC medications.
• Rule out medical causes for anxiety.
• Patient should have had routine complete physical within last year.
• Monitor vital signs during acute alcohol withdrawal; liver and kidney function; CBC with differential during long-term therapy.
• If discontinuing, taper dosage gradually (25% per week) and monitor for withdrawal symptoms.

Drug-Specific Patient Education
• Review symptoms specific to individual patient which drug potentially treats (symptoms of anxiety, panic, seizures, mania, tics, restless legs).
• Review dosing schedule until patient demonstrates a clear understanding of regimen.
• Discuss expected onset of action.
• Review most common side effects (drowsiness, fatigue,

ataxia) and encourage patient to report any side effects promptly.
• Warn against concurrent alcohol or CNS depressants.
• Caution patient about possible tolerance and/or psychological and physical dependence.
• Warn against abrupt discontinuation.
• Review possible withdrawal symptoms (see above under "Tolerance/Dependence")

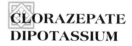

CLORAZEPATE DIPOTASSIUM

Apo-Clorazepate (CAN), Gen-Xene, Novo-Clopate (CAN), Tranxene

PREGNANCY CATEGORY D

C-IV controlled substance

Drug Classification: *Type:* anxiolytic; *Class:* 2-keto-benzodiazepine.

Mechanisms of Action
Benzodiazepines bind to specific receptor sites associated with the major inhibitory neurotransmitter in the brain, gamma-aminobutyric acid (GABA), thereby increasing the affinity of the receptor sites. While the exact mechanisms of action are not completely understood, inhibitory actions on neurons

within the limbic system, and on serotonergic (5-HT) and noradrenergic neurons within the brainstem, are responsible for the anxiolytic properties.

Indications
Relief of symptoms of anxiety. Adjunctive therapy in the management of partial seizures. Symptomatic relief of acute alcohol withdrawal.

Contraindications/Cautions
Contraindications: • hypersensitivity to benzodiazepines • psychoses, acute narrow-angle glaucoma, shock, coma, acute alcoholic intoxication • pregnancy (cleft lip or palate, inguinal hernia, cardiac defects, microcephaly, pyloric stenosis when used in first trimester; neonatal withdrawal syndrome reported in babies) • lactation.
Use cautiously with: • patients with history of alcohol or drug dependence or addiction • elderly or debilitated patients • patients with impaired liver or kidney function.

Dosage
Adult: 7.5–60 mg/d; may be given bid–qid.

Pediatric Adolescent: >6 y: 7.5–60 mg/d; >6 y: not recommended.

Geriatric: Initial dose 3.75 mg/d; adjust dose according to tolerance and remission of symptoms.

Dosage Forms: Tablets: 3.75, 7.5, 11.25, 15, 22.5 mg; Capsules 3.75, 7.5, 15 mg.

Pharmacokinetics
Absorption: from GI tract at rapid rate with rapid onset of action. *Distribution:* highly lipid soluble, crosses placenta, passes into breast milk. *Metabolism:* hepatic; $T_{1/2}$: 48–100 h. *Peak plasma level:* 6 h. *Steady state:* up to 2 wk. *Elimination:* urine.

Adverse Effects
CNS: Transient, mild drowsiness initially; sedation, fatigue, ataxia; confusion, depression, lethargy, stupor, apathy, lightheadedness, disorientation, dysarthria, headache, slurred speech, tremor, vertigo, diplopia, nystagmus, paradoxical excitatory reactions, anxiety, hallucinations, euphoria, difficulty in concentration, vivid dreams, psychomotor retardation increased muscle spasticity, insomnia, rage, sleep disturbances, minor changes in EEG patterns.
GI: Constipation, changes in salivation, nausea, anorexia, vomiting, difficulty in swallowing, elevations of blood enzymes—LDH, alkaline phosphatase, SGOT, SGPT;

hepatic dysfunction, jaundice.

CV: Bradycardia, tachycardia, hypertension and hypotension, palpitations, edema.

HEMATOLOGIC: Neutropenia, blood dyscrasias.

GU: Incontinence, urinary retention, changes in libido.

DERMATOLOGIC: Skin rashes.

TOLERANCE/DEPENDENCE: Some patients report a tolerance to the anxiolytic effects of benzodiazepines and require increased doses to maintain clinical remission. There is also a cross-tolerance among most of the benzodiazepines. Abrupt discontinuation, particularly of those with short half-lives, is associated with severe withdrawal symptoms seen only in patients who have taken high doses for long periods. Appearance of the syndrome may be delayed for 1–2 wk with benzodiazepines with very long half-lives. Commonly observed withdrawal symptoms in benzodiaz- epine withdrawal syndrome: anxiety, irritability, insomnia, fatigue, headache, muscle twitching or aching, tremor, shakiness, sweating, dizziness, concentration difficulties, nausea, anorexia, observable depression, depersonalization, derealization, increased sensory perception, abnormal perception or sensation of movement.

Clinically Important Drug–Drug Interactions

⇥ Decreased absorption with antacids.

⇥ Increased CNS depression with antihistamines, barbiturates and similarly acting drugs, cyclic antidepressants, alcohol, omeprazole.

⇥ Increased benzodiazepine level with cimetidine, disulfiram, erythromycin, estrogens, fluoxetine, isoniazid.

⇥ Decreased benzodiazepine levels with carbamazepine and, possibly, other anticonvulsants, theophyllines, ranitidine.

Nursing Considerations

Assessment

• Assess for any of the conditions listed under "Contraindications/Cautions" above.

• Assess for history of alcohol or drug dependence or abuse, use of concurrent prescribed or OTC medications.

• Patient should have had routine complete physical within last year.

• Monitor vital signs during acute alcohol withdrawal; liver and kidney function; CBC with differential during long-term therapy.

• If discontinuing, taper dosage gradually (25% per week) and monitor for withdrawal symptoms.

Drug-Specific Patient Education

• Review symptoms specific to individual patient which drug potentially treats (anxiety, alcohol withdrawal, panic, phobias, insomnia).
• Review dosing schedule until patient demonstrates a clear understanding of regimen.
• Discuss expected onset of action.
• Review most common side effects (drowsiness, fatigue, ataxia) and encourage patient to report any side effects promptly.
• Caution patient about possible tolerance and/or psychological and physical dependence.
• Warn against abrupt discontinuation.
• Review possible withdrawal symptoms (see above under "Tolerance/Dependence").

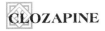

CLOZAPINE

Clozaril

PREGNANCY CATEGORY B

Drug Classification: *Type:* antipsychotic drug; *Class:* dopaminergic blocker.

Mechanisms of Action

Clozapine's mechanism of action is not fully understood. It blocks dopamine receptors in the brain and depresses the reticular activating system. It is anticholinergic, antihistaminic (H1), and alpha-adrenergic blocking. Clozapine produces fewer extrapyramidal effects than other antipsychotics.

Indications

Management of severely ill schizophrenic patients who fail to respond adequately to standard antipsychotic drug treatment.

Contraindications/Cautions

Contraindications: • allergy to clozapine • myeloproliferative disorders • history of clozapine-induced agranulocytosis or severe granulocytopenia • severe CNS depression • comatose states • history of seizure disorders • lactation.
Use cautiously with: • the presence of cardiovascular disease • prostate enlargement • narrow-angle glaucoma • pregnancy.

Dosage

Adult: Initially 25 mg PO qd or bid; then gradually continue to increase with daily dosage increments of 25–50 mg/d, if tolerated, to a dose of 300–450 mg/d by the end of 2 wk. Make subsequent dosage increments no more than once or twice weekly in increments not to exceed 100 mg. Do not exceed 900 mg/d. *Maintenance:* Maintain at the lowest effective dose needed to maintain remission of symptoms. *Discontinuation:* Gradual reduction of dose over a 2-wk period is preferred. If abrupt discontinuation is required, carefully monitor patient for signs of acute psychotic symptoms. *Reinitiation of treatment:* Follow initial dosage guidelines, using extreme care due to increased risk of severe adverse effects with reexposure.

Pediatric Adolescent: Safety and efficacy in children <16 y not established.

Dosage Forms: Tablets: 25 mg, 100 mg.

Pharmacokinetics

Absorption: well-absorbed from GI tract. *Distribution:* highly plasma protein-bound; crosses placenta and passes into breast milk. *Metabolism:* hepatic; $T_{1/2}$: 4–12 h; peak level: 1–6 h. *Elimination:* urine and feces.

Adverse Effects

CNS: Drowsiness, sedation, seizures, dizziness, syncope, headache, tremor, disturbed sleep, nightmares, restlessness, agitation, increased salivation, sweating.

CV: Tachycardia, hypotension, ECG changes, hypertension.

GI: Nausea, vomiting, constipation, abdominal discomfort, dry mouth.

GU: Urinary abnormalities.

HEMATOLOGIC: Leukopenia, granulocytopenia, agranulocytopenia.

OTHER: Fever, weight gain, rash.

Clinically Important Drug–Drug Interactions

⇇ Increased therapeutic and toxic effects of clozapine with cimetidine.

⇇ Decreased therapeutic effect of clozapine if taken with phenytoin, mephenytoin, ethotoin.

Nursing Considerations

Assessment

• Assess for any condition listed under "Contraindications/Cautions" above.

• Assess for history of alcohol or drug dependence or abuse, use of current prescribed or OTC medications.

• Complete physical exam: vital signs, orthostatic BP, intraocular pressure, ophthalmologic exam, CBC, urinalysis, liver and kidney function tests, EEG as appropriate.

• Administer only after patient has been tried on conventional antipsychotic drugs and found to be unresponsive to that drug therapy.

• Arrange for periodic monitoring of WBC weekly before treatment, during treatment, and for the 4 wk following the discontinuation of clozapine.
• Arrange to obtain clozapine through the Clozaril Patient Management System.
• Follow guidelines for discontinuation or reinstitution of the drug carefully.

Drug-Specific Patient Education
• Review the target symptoms that the drug potentially treats: relief of schizophrenic manifestations.
• Review the dosing schedule until patient demonstrates a clear understanding of regimen and the importance of continual use of drug.
• Review the most common side effects: drowsiness, dizziness, sedation, seizures; dizziness, faintness on arising; increased salivation; fast heart rate; constipation.
• Review the side effects patient should report promptly: lethargy, weakness, fever, sore throat, malaise, mouth ulcers, and "flu-like" symptoms.
• Caution patient that weekly blood tests are needed to determine safe dosage; dosage will be increased gradually to achieve most effective dose. Only 1 wk of medication can be dispensed at a time.
• Caution patient not to discontinue drug abruptly as serious side effects could occur.
• Caution patient to use some form of contraceptive and to avoid pregnancy while on this drug.
• Caution patient to avoid the use of alcohol and sleep-inducing or OTC drugs.

DESIPRAMINE HYDROCHLORIDE

••••••••••••••••••••••••••

Norpramin, Pertofrane

PREGNANCY CATEGORY C

Drug Classification: *Type:* Antidepressant; *Class:* tricyclic (TCA); *Subclass:* secondary amine.

Mechanisms of Action
Presynaptic reuptake inhibition of neurotransmitters norepinephrine and serotonin (antidepressant efficacy is thought to be mediated by these actions). Postsynaptic blockade of histaminic, muscarinic, and noradrenergic alpha-one and alpha-two receptors (some of the undesirable side effects are thought to be mediated by these actions).

Indications
Relief of symptoms of depression (endogenous depression most responsive).

Relief of symptoms of anxiety
and panic disorders.
Control of chronic pain.

Contraindications/Cautions

Contraindications: • hypersensitivity to any tricyclic drug
• concomitant therapy with an
MAO inhibitor • ECT with
coadministration of TCAs • recent MI • myelography within
previous 24 h or scheduled
within 48 h.

Use cautiously with: • preexisting CV disorders • seizure
disorders • hyperthyroidism
• angle-closure glaucoma • increased intraocular pressure
• urinary retention • ureteral
or urethral spasm • impaired
hepatic or renal function
• bipolar patients shifting to
hypomanic or manic phase
• elective surgery • pregnancy
• lactation.

Dosage

Adult: Typical starting dose 50
mg qhs. Can be administered
once a day, usually at hs, or in divided doses if patient has side
effects due to high peak levels.
Increase by 50 mg q 3–4 d as
side effects allow. Usual maintenance dose 150–300 mg/d. Extreme dose 300 mg qd. Earliest
onset of action in 2–5 d. Consider drug trial a failure if patient
has been on maximal dose for
4–6 wk without response. Limit
potentially suicidal patients' access to drug.

Pediatric Adolescent: Not recommended in children <12 y.

Geriatric: Initially 10 mg/d. Adjust dose according to tolerance and blood level.

Dosage Forms: Tablets: 10, 25,
50, 75, 100, 150 mg.

Blood Levels: Draw only to assess
compliance; to confirm rapid or
slow metabolizers; to document adequate drug trial. Patients with a level of desipramine greater than 125
ng/ml may improve more than
those below that level. Range of
therapeutic levels is considered
to be 150–300; levels should be
drawn when any dose has
reached steady state (5–7 d)
and 10–14 h after last dose.

Pharmacokinetics

Absorption: from GI tract
rapidly and completely. *Distribution:* highly lipophilic and
largely protein bound; crosses
blood–brain barrier and placenta and enters breast milk.
Metabolism: hepatic; $T_{1/2}$:
48–72 h. *Elimination:* urine.
Steady state: 5–7 d.

Adverse Effects

Adult Use

   CNS: Sedation and anticholinergic effects—dry mouth,

blurred vision, disturbance of accommodation for near vision, mydriasis, increased intraocular pressure; confusion, disturbed concentration, hallucinations, disorientation, decreased memory, feelings of unreality, delusions, anxiety, nervousness, restlessness, agitation, panic, insomnia, nightmares, hypomania, mania, exacerbation of psychosis, drowsiness, weakness, fatigue, headache, numbness, tingling, paresthesias of extremities, discoordination, motor hyperactivity, akathisia, ataxia, tremors, peripheral neuropathy, extrapyramidal symptoms, seizures, speech blockage, dysarthria, tinnitus, altered EEG.

GI: Dry mouth, constipation, paralytic ileus, nausea, vomiting, anorexia, epigastric distress, diarrhea, flatulence, dysphagia, peculiar taste, increased salivation, stomatitis, glossitis, parotid swelling, abdominal cramps, black tongue, hepatitis.

CV: Orthostatic hypotension, hypertension, syncope, tachycardia, palpitations, MI, arrhythmias, heart block, precipitation of CHF, stroke.

HEMATOLOGIC: Bone marrow depression, including agranulocytosis; eosinophilia, purpura, thrombocytopenia.

GU: Urinary retention, delayed micturition, dilation of the urinary tract, gynecomastia, testicular swelling in men; breast enlargement, menstrual irregularity, and galactorrhea in women; increased or decreased libido; impotence.

HYPERSENSITIVITY: Skin rash, pruritus, vasculitis, petechiae, photosensitization, edema (generalized, facial, tongue), drug fever.

ENDOCRINE: Elevated or depressed blood sugar, elevated prolactin levels, inappropriate ADH secretion.

WITHDRAWAL: Abrupt discontinuation of prolonged therapy: nausea, headache, vertigo, nightmares, malaise.

OTHER: Nasal congestion, excessive appetite, weight gain or loss; sweating (paradoxical effect in a drug with prominent anticholinergic effects), alopecia, lacrimation, hyperthermia, flushing, chills.

Clinically Important Drug–Drug Interactions

⊰ Increased sedation with alcohol, antihistamines, antipsychotics, barbiturates, chloral hydrate, and other sedatives.

⊰ Increased hypotension with alpha-methyldopa, beta-adrenergic blockers, clonidine, diuretics, low-potency antipsychotics.

⚜ Additive cardiotoxicity with quinidine and other class II antiarrhythmics, thioridazine, mesoridazine, pimozide.

⚜ Additive anticholinergic toxicity with antihistamines, antiparkinsonians, low-potency antipsychotics, especially thioridazine, over-the-counter sleeping medications, gastrointestinal antispasmodics and antidiarrheals.

⚜ TCAs may increase the effects of warfarin and block the effects of guanethidine.

⚜ Increased sympathomimetic (especially alpha-adrenergic) effects of direct-acting sympathomimetic drugs (norepinephrine, epinephrine).

⚜ Decreased effects of indirect-acting sympathomimetic drugs (ephedrine).

⚜ Increased levels and possible delirium with disulfiram.

Note: MAOIs and TCAs have been used successfully in some patients who are resistant to therapy with single agents; however, hyperpyretic crises, severe convulsions, hypertensive episodes, and deaths can occur when MAOIs are given with TCAs.

Nursing Considerations

Assessment

• Assess for any of the conditions listed under "Contraindications/Cautions" above.

• Assess for ETOH or drug use/abuse and for concomitant prescribed and/or OTC medications.

• Assess for suicidal ideation.

• Complete physical exam: vital signs, EKG for patients 40 y or older, CBC with differential, thyroid function, liver function, BUN, creatinine, weight changes, I & O, vision; sexual interest, function, and activity.

Drug-Specific Patient Education

• Review target symptoms that drug potentially treats: disruptions in sleep, appetite, concentration, energy, mood; anhedonia; interest; motivation; initiative.

• Review dosing schedule until patient demonstrates a clear understanding of regimen.

• Discuss expected lag period (3–4 wk) before therapeutic effects can be anticipated.

• Review most common side effects: dry mouth, constipation, dizziness, urinary hesitancy, headache, nausea, sedation, or agitation, and encourage patient to report any side effects promptly.

• Caution patient against abrupt discontinuation without consulting prescriber. Abrupt discontinuation may cause withdrawal symptoms (cholinergic rebound, malaise, chills, coryza, muscle aches, agitation, insomnia) or rapid reemergence of depressive symptoms.

• Caution patient about ETOH or drug use.

DEXTROAMPHE-TAMINE SULFATE

••••••••••••••••••••••••••••

Dexedrine

PREGNANCY CATEGORY C

C-II controlled substance

Drug Classification: *Type:* CNS stimulant *Class:* Amphetamine.

Mechanisms of Action

Acts in the CNS to release norepinephrine from nerve terminals; in higher doses also releases dopamine; suppresses appetite; increases alertness, elevates mood; often improves physical performance, especially when fatigue and sleep-deprivation have caused impairment. Efficacy in hyperkinetic syndrome; attention-deficit disorders in children appears paradoxical and is not understood.

Indications

Narcolepsy.

Abnormal behavioral syndrome in children (attention deficit disorder, hyperkinetic syndrome) as part of treatment program that includes psychological, social, educational measures.

Contraindications/Cautions

Contraindications: • hypersensitivity to sympathomimetic amines, tartrazine (in preparations marketed as Dexedrine) • advanced arteriosclerosis • symptomatic cardiovascular disease • moderate to severe hypertension • hyperthyroidism • glaucoma • agitated states • history of drug abuse • pregnancy • lactation.

Use cautiously with: • mild hypertension • suicidal ideation.

Dosage

Adult: Start with 10 mg/d PO in divided doses; increase in increments of 10 mg/d at weekly intervals. If adverse reactions (insomnia, anorexia) occur, reduce dose. Usual dosage is 560 mg/d PO in divided doses. Give first dose on awakening, additional doses (1 or 2) q 4–6 h; long-acting forms can be given once a day.

Pediatric Adolescent: *Narcolepsy:* 6–12 y: condition is rare in children <12 y; when it does occur, initial dose is 5 mg/d PO. Increase in increments of 5 mg at weekly intervals until optimal response is obtained. ≥12 y: Use adult dosage.

Attention deficit disorder: <3 y: Not recommended. 3–5 y: 2.5 mg/d PO. Increase in increments of 2.5 mg/d at weekly intervals until optimal response is obtained. ≥6 y: 5 mg PO qd–bid. Increase in increments of 5 mg/d at weekly intervals until optimal response is obtained. Dosage will rarely exceed 40 mg/d. Give first dose on awakening, additional doses (1 or 2) q 4–6 h. Long-acting forms may be used for once-a-day dosage.

Dosage Forms: Tablets: 5, 10 mg; Sustained release capsules: 5, 10, 15 mg.

Pharmacokinetics

Absorption: rapidly from the GI tract. *Distribution:* widely distributed, including brain tissue; crosses placenta, passes into breast milk. *Metabolism:* hepatic; $T_{1/2}$: 10–30 h. *Peak levels:* 1–5 h. *Duration:* 8–10 h. *Elimination:* urine.

Adverse Effects

CV: Palpitations, tachycardia, hypertension.

CNS: Overstimulation, restlessness, dizziness, insomnia, dyskinesia, euphoria, dysphoria, tremor, headache, psychotic episodes.

GI: Dry mouth, unpleasant taste, diarrhea, constipation, anorexia and weight loss.

DERMATOLOGIC: Urticaria.

GU: Impotence, changes in libido.

ENDOCRINE: Reversible eleva-

tions in serum thyroxine with heavy use.

OTHER: Tolerance, psychological dependence, social disability with abuse.

Clinically Important Drug–Drug Interactions

⊞ Hypertensive crisis and increased CNS effects of dextroamphetamine if given within 14 d of monoamine oxidase inhibitors (MAOIs)—DO NOT GIVE DEXTROAMPHETAMINE to patients who are taking or who have recently taken MAOIs.
⊞ Increased duration of effects of dextroamphetamine taken with urinary alkalinizers (acetazolamide, sodium bicarbonate), furazolidone.
⊞ Decreased effects of dextroamphetamine taken with urinary acidifiers.
⊞ Decreased efficacy of antihypertensive drugs (guanethidine) given with amphetamines.

Nursing Considerations

Assessment
• Assess for any conditions listed under "Contraindications/Cautions" above.
• Assess for any history or alcohol or drug dependence or abuse, current use of prescribed or OTC medications.
• Complete physical exam: vital signs, ophthalmologic

exam (tonometry), thyroid function tests, blood and urine glucose.

• Assess for proper diagnosis before administering to children for behavioral syndromes: drug should not be used until other causes/concomitants of abnormal behavior (learning disability, EEG abnormalities, neurological deficits) are ruled out.

• Assess growth of children on long-term therapy; interrupt drug dosage periodically in children being treated for behavioral disorders to determine if symptoms recur at an intensity that warrants continued drug therapy.

Drug-Specific Patient Education

• Review the target symptoms that the drug potentially treats: hyperactivity, attention deficit, sleep problems.

• Review the dosing schedule until patient and/or significant other demonstrates a clear understanding of drug regimen, including taking drug early in the day to avoid nighttime sleep disturbances.

• Review the most common side effects: nervousness, restlessness, dizziness, insomnia, impaired thinking, headache, loss of appetite, dry mouth.

• Review the side effects patient should report promptly: nervousness, insomnia, dizziness, palpitations, anorexia, GI disturbances.

• Caution patient to avoid pregnancy while on this drug; use of barrier contraceptives is advised.

• Caution patient to avoid alcohol and sleep-inducing or OTC preparations.

DIAZEPAM

Apo-Diazepam (CAN), Diazemuls (CAN), Valium, Valrelease, Vivol (CAN), Zetran

PREGNANCY CATEGORY D

C-IV controlled substance

Drug Classification: *Type:* anxiolytic, antiepileptic, sedative-hypnotic, skeletal muscle relaxant; *Class:* 2-keto-benzodiazepine.

Mechanisms of Action

Benzodiazepines bind to specific receptor sites associated with the major inhibitory neurotransmitter in the brain, gamma-aminobutyric acid (GABA), thereby increasing the affinity of the receptor sites. While the exact mechanisms of action are not completely understood, inhibitory actions on neurons within the limbic system, and on serotonergic (5-HT) and noradrenergic neurons within the brainstem, are responsible for the anxiolytic properties, and actions on cortical neurons may be responsible for the antiepileptic effects.

Indications

Relief of symptoms of anxiety.

Symptomatic relief of acute alcohol withdrawal; adjunct relief for reflex skeletal muscle spasm or spasticity; antiepileptic.

Relief of panic symptoms and phobias.

Treatment of generalized anxiety disorder; insomnia; akathisia.

Contraindications/Cautions

Contraindications: • hypersensitivity to benzodiazepines • psychoses, acute narrow-angle glaucoma, shock, coma, acute alcoholic intoxication • pregnancy (cleft lip or palate, inguinal hernia, cardiac defects, microcephaly, pyloric stenosis when used in first trimester; neonatal withdrawal syndrome reported in babies) • lactation.

Use cautiously with: • patients with a history of alcohol or drug dependence or addiction • elderly or debilitated patients • patients with impaired liver or kidney function.

Dosage

Adult: Usual range (oral and parenteral): 2–60 mg/d; oral may be given bid–qid.

Pediatric Adolescent: 0.2–10 mg/d

Geriatric: Initial dose 1 mg/d;

adjust dose according to tolerance and remission of symptoms.

Dosage Forms: Tablets: 2, 5, 10 mg; Capsules (extended release): 15 mg; Parenteral: 5 mg/ml.

Pharmacokinetics

Absorption: from GI tract rapidly and completely with rapid onset of action. *Distribution:* highly lipid soluble. *Metabolism:* hepatic; $T_{1/2}$: 30–100 h. *Peak plasma level:* 1–3 h. *Steady state:* up to 2 wk. *Elimination:* urine.

Adverse Effects

CNS: Transient, mild drowsiness initially; sedation, fatigue, ataxia; confusion, depression, lethargy, stupor, apathy, light-headedness, disorientation, dysarthria, headache, slurred speech, tremor, vertigo, diplopia, nystagmus, paradoxical excitatory reactions, anxiety, hallucinations, euphoria, difficulty in concentration, vivid dreams, psychomotor retardation increased muscle spasticity, insomnia, rage, sleep disturbances, minor changes in EEG patterns.

GI: Constipation, changes in salivation, nausea, anorexia, vomiting, difficulty in swallowing, elevations of blood enzymes—LDH, alkaline phosphatase, SGOT, SGPT; hepatic dysfunction, jaundice.

CV: Bradycardia, tachycardia, hypertension and hypotension, palpitations, edema.

HEMATOLOGIC: Neutropenia, blood dyscrasias.

GU: Incontinence, urinary retention, changes in libido.

DERMATOLOGIC: Skin rashes.

TOLERANCE/DEPENDENCE: Some patients report a tolerance to the anxiolytic effects of benzodiazepines and require increased doses to maintain clinical remission. There is also a cross-tolerance among most of the benzodiazepines. Abrupt discontinuation, particularly of those with short half-lives, is associated with severe withdrawal symptoms seen only in patients who have taken high doses for long periods. Appearance of the syndrome may be delayed for 1–2 wk with benzodiazepines with very long half-lives. Commonly observed withdrawal symptoms in benzodiazepine withdrawal syndrome: anxiety, irritability, insomnia, fatigue, headache, muscle twitching or aching, tremor, shakiness, sweating, dizziness, concentration difficulties, nausea, anorexia, observable depression, depersonalization, derealization, increased sensory perception, abnormal perception or sensation of movement.

Clinically Important Drug–Drug Interactions

⧧ Decreased absorption with antacids.

⧧ Increased CNS depression with antihistamines, barbiturates and similarly acting drugs, cyclic antidepressants, alcohol, omeprazole.

⧧ Increased benzodiazepine level with cimetidine, disulfiram, erythromycin, estrogens, fluoxetine, isoniazid.

⧧ Decreased benzodiazepine levels with carbamazepine and, possibly, other anticonvulsants, theophyllines, ranitidine.

Nursing Considerations

Assessment

• Assess for any of the conditions listed under "Contraindications/Cautions" above.

• Assess for history of alcohol or drug dependence or abuse, use of concurrent prescribed or OTC medications.

• Patient should have had routine complete physical within last year.

• Monitor liver and kidney function; CBC with differential during long-term therapy.

• If discontinuing, taper dosage gradually (25% per week), and monitor for withdrawal symptoms.

Drug-Specific Patient Education

• Review symptoms specific to

individual patient which drug potentially treats (anxiety, panic, phobias, insomnia).
• Review dosing schedule until patient demonstrates a clear understanding of regimen.
• Discuss expected onset of action.
• Review most common side effects (drowsiness, fatigue, ataxia) and encourage patient to report any side effects promptly.
• Caution patient about possible tolerance and dependence.
• Warn against abrupt discontinuation.
• Review possible withdrawal symptoms (see above under "Tolerance/Dependence").

DIPHEN-HYDRAMINE HYDROCHLORIDE

••••••••••••••••••••••••••

Oral prescription preparations: Benadryl
Parenteral preparations: Benadryl, Benahist, Benoject, Diphenacen

PREGNANCY CATEGORY B

Drug Classification: *Type:* sedative, antiparkinsonian; *Class:* antihistamine; *Subclass:* ethanolamine.

Mechanisms of Action
Competitively blocks the effects of histamine at H1 receptor sites; has atropine-like, antipruritic and sedative effects.

Indications
Parkinsonism (including drug-induced Parkinsonism and extrapyramidal reactions) in the elderly intolerant of more potent agents, for milder forms of the disorder in other age groups, and in combination with centrally acting anticholinergic antiparkinsonism drugs.

Contraindications/Cautions
Contraindications: • allergy to any antihistamines • third trimester of pregnancy • lactation.
Use cautiously with:
• narrow-angle glaucoma
• stenosing peptic ulcer • symptomatic prostatic hypertrophy
• asthmatic attack • bladder neck obstruction • pyloroduodenal obstruction • pregnancy.

Dosage
Adult: *Oral:* 25–50 mg q 4–6 h. *Parenteral:* 10–50 mg IV or deep IM; up to 100 mg if required. Maximum daily dose is 400 mg.

Pediatric Adolescent: >10 kg, 20 lb: *Oral:* 12.5–25 mg tid–qid or 5 mg/kg/d or 150 mg/m²/d. Maximum daily dose 300 mg.

Parenteral: 5 mg/kg/d or 150 mg/m²/d IV or by deep IM injection. Maximum daily dose is 300 mg divided into 4 doses.

Geriatric: More likely to cause dizziness, sedation, syncope, toxic confusional states, and hypotension in elderly patients>use with caution.

Dosage Forms: Tablets: 25, 50 mg; Capsules: 25, 50 mg; Elixir: 12.5 mg/5 ml; Syrup: 12.5 mg/5 ml; Injection: 10 mg/ml, 50 mg/ml.

Pharmacokinetics

Absorption: rapidly from the GI tract and muscle. *Distribution:* widely distributed; crosses placenta and passes into breast milk. *Metabolism:* hepatic; $T_{1/2}$: 2.5–7 h. *Peak levels:* 1–4 h. *Duration:* 4–8 h. *Elimination:* urine.

Adverse Effects

CV: Hypotension, palpitations, bradycardia, tachycardia, extrasystoles.

HEMATOLOGIC: Hemolytic anemia, hypoplastic anemia, thrombocytopenia, leukopenia, agranulocytosis, pancytopenia.

CNS: Drowsiness, sedation, dizziness, disturbed coordination, fatigue, confusion, restlessness, excitation, nervousness, tremor, headache, blurred vision, diplopia.

GI: Epigastric distress, anorexia, increased appetite and weight gain, nausea, vomiting, diarrhea, or constipation.

GU: Urinary frequency, dysuria, urinary retention, early menses, decreased libido, impotence.

RESPIRATORY: Thickening of bronchial secretions, chest tightness, wheezing, nasal stuffiness, dry mouth, dry nose, dry throat, sore throat.

OTHER: Urticaria, rash, anaphylactic shock, photosensitivity, excessive perspiration.

Clinically Important Drug–Drug Interactions

⊄ Possible increased and prolonged anticholinergic effects if taken with MAOIs.

Nursing Considerations

Assessment
• Assess patient for any conditions listed under "Contraindications/Cautions" above.
• Assess for any history of drug abuse or dependence, current use of prescribed or OTC medications
• Complete physical exam: vital signs, vision exam, CBC with differential.

Drug-Specific Patient Education
• Review the target symptoms the drug potentially treats: drooling, lack of coordination,

shuffling, speech impairment
• Review the dosing schedule until patient demonstrates a clear understanding of drug regimen.
• Review the most common side effects: dizziness, sedation, drowsiness, epigastric distress, diarrhea or constipation, dry mouth, thickening of bronchial secretions, dryness of nasal mucosa.
• Review the side effects patient should report promptly: difficulty breathing, hallucinations, tremors, loss of coordination, unusual bleeding or bruising, visual disturbances, irregular heartbeat.
• Caution patient to avoid alcohol and sleep-inducing or OTC medications.

DIVALPROEX SODIUM

• •

Depakote, Epival (CAN)

PREGNANCY CATEGORY D

Drug Classification: *Type:* anticonvulsant.

Mechanisms of Action
Mechanism of action is not completely understood; antiepileptic activity may be related to the metabolism of the inhibitory neurotransmitter, gamma-aminobutyric acid (GABA). Divalproex sodium is a compound containing equal proportions of valproic acid and sodium valproate.

Indications
Sole and adjunctive therapy in simple (petit mal) and complex absence seizures.
Adjunctive therapy in patients with multiple seizure types including absence seizures.
Treatment of manic episodes associated with bipolar disease.
Unlabeled uses: Sole and adjunctive therapy in atypical absence, myoclonic and grand mal seizures, and possibly effective therapy in atonic, complex partial, elementary partial, and infantile spasm seizures; prophylaxis for recurrent febrile seizures in children.

Contraindications/Cautions
Contraindications: hypersensitivity to valproic acid • hepatic disease or significant hepatic dysfunction.
Use cautiously with: • children <18 mo • children <2 y, especially those receiving multiple antiepileptic drugs, those with congenital metabolic disorders, those with severe seizures accompanied by severe mental retardation, those with organic brain disorders • pregnancy • lactation.

Dosage

Adult: Dosage is expressed as valproic acid equivalents. Initial dose is 15 mg/kg/d PO, increasing at 1 wk intervals by 5–10 mg/kg/d until seizures are controlled or side effects preclude further increases. Maximum recommended dosage is 60 mg/kg/d. If total dose >250 mg/d, give in divided doses.

Pediatric: Use extreme caution. Fatal hepatotoxicity has occurred. Children <2 y are especially susceptible. Monitor all children carefully.

Dosage Forms: Capsules: 250 mg; Syrup: 250 mg/5 ml; Delayed release tablets: 125 mg, 250 mg, 500 mg; Sprinkle capsules: 125 mg.

Blood Levels: Therapeutic serum levels—usually 50–100 mcg/ml.

Pharmacokinetics

Absorption: rapid from the GI tract. *Distribution:* widely distributed; crosses blood brain barrier; crosses placenta and passes into breast milk. *Metabolism:* hepatic; $T_{1/2}$: 6–16 h. *Elimination:* urine and feces.

Adverse Effects

GI: Nausea, vomiting, indigestion, diarrhea, abdominal cramps, constipation, anorexia with weight loss, increased appetite with weight gain.

HEMATOLOGIC: Slight elevations in SGOT, SGPT, LDH; increases in serum bilirubin, abnormal changes in other liver function tests, hepatic failure, altered bleeding time; thrombocytopenia; bruising; hematoma formation; frank hemorrhage; relative lymphocytosis; hypofibrinogenemia; leukopenia, eosinophilia, anemia, bone marrow suppression.

CNS: Sedation, tremor (may be dose-related), emotional upset, depression, psychosis, aggression, hyperactivity, behavioral deterioration, weakness.

DERMATOLOGIC: Transient increases in hair loss; skin rash; petechiae.

GU: Irregular menses, secondary amenorrhea.

Clinically Important Drug–Drug Interactions

⧐ Increased serum phenobarbital, primidone levels if taken concurrently.

⧐ Complex interactions with phenytoin; breakthrough seizures have occurred with the combination of valproic acid and phenytoin.

⧐ Increased valproic acid serum levels and toxicity if given concurrently with salicylates.

⧐ Decreased valproic acid effects if given concurrently with carbamazepine.

≠ Decreased serum levels of valproic acid if given concurrently with charcoal.

Nursing Considerations

Assessment
• Assess for any condtions listed under "Contraindications/Cautions" above.
• Assess for history of alcohol or drug abuse or dependence, current use of prescribed or OTC medications.
• Complete physical exam: vital signs; CBC and differential, bleeding time tests, hepatic function tests, serum ammonia level, exocrine pancreatic function tests, EEG.
• Assess liver function tests frequently—arrange to discontinue drug immediately in the presence of significant hepatic dysfunction, suspected or apparent; hepatic dysfunction has progressed in spite of drug discontinuation.
• Assess for patient platelet counts, bleeding time determination before initiating therapy, at periodic intervals during therapy, and prior to surgery.
• Monitor patient carefully for signs of clotting defect—bruising, blood-tinged toothbrush, etc. Arrange to discontinue drug if there is evidence of hemorrhage, bruising, or disorder of hemostasis.

• Assess ammonia levels and arrange to discontinue drug in the presence of clinically significant elevation in levels.
• Assess for frequent monitoring of serum levels of valproic acid and other antiepileptic drugs given concomitantly, especially during the first few weeks of therapy. Arrange to adjust dosage as appropriate on the basis of these data and clinical response.

Drug-Specific Patient Education
• Review the target symptoms the drug potentially treats: frequency and intensity of seizures, manic episodes.
• Review the dosing schedule until patient demonstrates clear understanding of drug regimen.
• Review the most common side effects: drowsiness, GI upset, transient increase in hair loss.
• Review the side effects patient should report promptly: bruising, pink stain on the toothbrush, yellowing of the skin or eyes, pale-colored feces, skin rash, pregnancy.
• Caution patient to avoid pregnancy, use of barrier contraceptives is advised.
• Caution patient not to discontinue drug abruptly as serious side effects could occur.
• Caution diabetic patients that drug may interfere with urine tests for ketones.

• Caution patient to avoid alcohol and sleep-inducing or OTC medications.

DOXEPIN HYDROCHLORIDE

••••••••••••••••••••••••••••

Novo-Doxepin (CAN), Sinequan, Adapin, Triadapin (CAN)

PREGNANCY CATEGORY C

Drug Classification: *Type:* Antidepressant; *Class:* tricyclic (TCA); *Subclass:* tertiary amine.

Mechanisms of Action

Presynaptic reuptake inhibition of neurotransmitters norepinephrine and serotonin (antidepressant efficacy is thought to be mediated by these actions). Postsynaptic blockade of histaminic, muscarinic, and noradrenergic alpha-one and alpha-two receptors (some of the undesirable side effects are thought to be mediated by these actions).

Indications

Relief of symptoms of depression (endogenous depression most responsive); sedative effects may help when depression is associated with anxiety and sleep disturbance. *Unlabeled uses:* relief of symptoms of anxiety.

Contraindications/Cautions

Contraindications: • hypersensitivity to any tricyclic drug • concomitant therapy with an MAO inhibitor • ECT with coadministration of TCAs • recent MI • myelography within previous 24 h or scheduled within 48 h.

Use cautiously with: • preexisting CV disorders, especially cardiac conduction system disease • seizure disorders • hyperthyroidism • angle-closure glaucoma • increased intraocular pressure • urinary retention • ureteral or urethral spasm • impaired hepatic or renal function • bipolar patients shifting to hypomanic or manic phase • elective surgery • pregnancy • lactation.

Dosage

Adult: Typical starting dose 25 mg qhs. Usual maintenance dose 150–300 mg/d. Earliest onset of action in 2–5 d. Consider drug trial a failure if patient has been on maximal dose for 4–6 wk without response. Limit potentially suicidal patients' access to drug.

Pediatric Adolescent: Not recommended in children <12 y.

Geriatric: Initially 25 mg/d. Adjust dose according to tolerance and blood level.

Dosage Forms: Capsules: 10, 25, 50, 75, 100, 150 mg.

Blood Levels: Draw only to assess compliance; to confirm rapid or slow metabolizers; to document adequate drug trial. Range of therapeutic level is 100–250 ng/ml; levels should be drawn when any dose has reached steady state (5–7 d) and 10–14 h after last dose.

Pharmacokinetics

Absorption: from GI tract rapidly and completely. *Distribution:* highly lipophilic and largely protein bound; crosses blood–brain barrier and placenta and enters breast milk. *Metabolism:* hepatic; $T_{1/2}$: 8–25 h. *Elimination:* urine. *Steady state:* 5–7 d.

Adverse Effects

Adult Use

CNS: Sedation and anticholinergic effects—dry mouth, blurred vision, disturbance of accommodation for near vision, mydriasis, increased intraocular pressure; confusion, disturbed concentration, hallucinations, disorientation, decreased memory, feelings of unreality, delusions, anxiety, nervousness, restlessness, agitation, panic, insomnia, nightmares, hypomania, mania, exacerbation of psychosis, drowsiness, weakness, fatigue, headache, numbness, tingling, paresthesias of extremities, discoordination, motor hyperactivity, akathisia, ataxia, tremors, peripheral neuropathy, extrapyramidal symptoms, seizures, speech blockage, dysarthria, tinnitus, altered EEG.

GI: Dry mouth, constipation, paralytic ileus, nausea, vomiting, anorexia, epigastric distress, diarrhea, flatulence, dysphagia, peculiar taste, increased salivation, stomatitis, glossitis, parotid swelling, abdominal cramps, black tongue, hepatitis.

CV: Orthostatic hypotension, hypertension, syncope, tachycardia, palpitations, MI, arrhythmias, heart block, precipitation of CHF, stroke.

HEMATOLOGIC: Bone marrow depression, including agranulocytosis; eosinophilia, purpura, thrombocytopenia.

GU: Urinary retention, delayed micturition, dilation of the urinary tract, gynecomastia, testicular swelling in men; breast enlargement, menstrual irregularity, and galactorrhea in women; increased or decreased libido; impotence.

HYPERSENSITIVITY: Skin rash, pruritus, vasculitis, petechiae, photosensitization, edema (generalized, facial, tongue), drug fever.

ENDOCRINE: Elevated or depressed blood sugar, elevated prolactin levels, inappropriate ADH secretion.

WITHDRAWAL: Abrupt discontinuation of prolonged therapy: nausea, headache, vertigo, nightmares, malaise.

OTHER: Nasal congestion, excessive appetite, weight gain or loss; sweating (paradoxical effect in a drug with prominent anticholinergic effects), alopecia, lacrimation, hyperthermia, flushing, chills.

Clinically Important Drug–Drug Interactions

Increased sedation with alcohol, antihistamines, antipsychotics, barbiturates, chloral hydrate, and other sedatives.
Increased hypotension with alpha-methyldopa, beta-adrenergic blockers, clonidine, diuretics, low-potency antipsychotics.
Additive cardiotoxicity with quinidine and other class II antiarrhythmics, thioridazine, mesoridazine, pimozide.
Additive anticholinergic toxicity with antihistamines, antiparkinsonians, low-potency antipsychotics, especially thioridazine, over-the-counter sleeping medications, gastrointestinal antispasmodics and antidiarrheals.
TCAs may increase the effects of warfarin and block the effects of guanethidine.
Increased sympathomimetic (especially alpha-adrenergic) effects of direct-acting sympathomimetic drugs (norepinephrine, epinephrine).
Decreased effects of indirect-acting sympathomimetic drugs (ephedrine).
Increased levels and possible delirium with disulfiram.

Note: MAOIs and TCAs have been used successfully in some patients who are resistant to therapy with single agents; however, hyperpyretic crises, severe convulsions, hypertensive episodes, and deaths can occur when MAOIs are given with TCAs.

Nursing Considerations

Assessment

• Assess for any of the conditions listed under "Contraindications/Cautions" above.
• Assess for ETOH or drug use/abuse and for concomitant prescribed and/or OTC medications.
• Complete physical exam; vital signs, EKG for patients 40 y or older, CBC with differential, thyroid function, liver function, BUN, creatinine, weight changes, I & O, vision; sexual interest, function, and activity.

Drug-Specific Patient Education

• Review target symptoms that drug potentially treats: disrup-

tions in sleep, appetite, concentration, energy, mood; anhedonia; interest; motivation; initiative.
• Review dosing schedule until patient demonstrates a clear understanding of regimen.
• Discuss expected lag period (3–4 wk) before therapeutic effects can be anticipated.
• Review most common side effects: dry mouth, constipation, dizziness, urinary hesitancy, headache, nausea, sedation, or agitation, and encourage patient to report any side effects promptly.
• Caution patient against abrupt discontinuation without consulting prescriber. Abrupt discontinuation may cause withdrawal symptoms (cholinergic rebound, malaise, chills, coryza, muscle aches, agitation, insomnia) or rapid reemergence of depressive symptoms.
• Caution patient about ETOH or drug use.

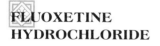

FLUOXETINE HYDROCHLORIDE

• •

Prozac

PREGNANCY CATEGORY B

Drug Classification: *Type:* specific serotonin reuptake inhibitor (SSRI) antidepressant; *Class:* phenylpropylamine derivative.

Mechanisms of Action
Antidepressant activity associated with presynaptic reuptake of serotonin; no significant effects on norepinephrine, dopamine, or on adrenergic, histaminergic, muscarinic, and serotonergic receptors.

Indications
Treatment of depression, dysthymia, eating disorders, obsessive-compulsive disorder, panic, premature ejaculation, posttraumatic stress disorder, premenstrual dysphoric disorder.

Contraindications/Cautions
Contraindications: • hypersensitivity to fluoxetine
• pregnancy • lactation.
Use cautiously with: • impaired hepatic or renal function • diabetes mellitus
• may precipitate mania.

Dosage
Adult: 10–80 mg/d. May be given qd, usually in a.m. Earliest onset of action within 2–5 d. Consider drug trial a failure if patient has been on maximum recommended dose for 4–6 wk without response.

Pediatric Adolescent: Start at one-half the adult dose and increase slowly and cautiously.

Geriatric: Start at one-half the adult dose and increase slowly and cautiously.

Dosage Forms: Capsules: 10, 20 mg; Liquid: 20 mg/5 ml.

Pharmacokinetics

Absorption: from the GI tract; reaches peak plasma levels in 4–8 h. *Distribution:* 94.5% protein-bound; crosses placenta, enters breast milk. *Metabolism:* hepatic; $T_{1/2}$: 2–3 d. *Steady state:* 2–3 wk. *Elimination:* urine and feces.

Adverse Effects

CNS: Headaches, nervousness, insomnia, drowsiness, anxiety, tremor, dizziness, fatigue, sedation, sensation disturbance, decreased libido, light-headedness, decreased concentration.

GI: Nausea, diarrhea, dry mouth, anorexia, dyspepsia, constipation, abdominal pain, vomiting, taste change, flatulence, gastroenteritis.

SKIN: Excessive sweating, rash, pruritus.

BODY AS A WHOLE: Asthenia, viral infection, chest and limb pain, fever.

RESPIRATORY: Flu-like syndrome, pharyngitis, nasal congestion, sinusitis.

CV: Hot flashes, palpitations.

MUSCULOSKELETAL: Back, joint, and muscle pain.

GU: Painful menstruation, sexual dysfunction.

SPECIAL SENSES: Visual disturbance.

Clinically Important Drug–Drug Interactions

♯ Note: Because of the prolonged elimination of fluoxetine and its metabolite, norfluoxetine (2–3 wk), the potential for drug–drug interactions exists even after fluoxetine therapy is discontinued.

♯ Fluoxetine increases plasma levels of tricyclics, trazodone, and benzodiazepines.

♯ Decreases therapeutic effects of cyproheptadine.

♯ Toxic reactions or serotonin syndrome may occur with MAOIs or L-tryptophan.

♯ May change levels of carbamazepine, lithium, and antipsychotics.

♯ May decrease efficacy of buspirone and may precipitate EPS.

Nursing Considerations

Assessment

• Assess for any of the conditions listed in "Contraindications/Cautions" above.

• Assess for concurrent prescription, OTC, or illegal drug use/abuse and ETOH use/abuse, risk of suicide, and limit drug access to potentially suicidal patients.

• Complete physical, vital signs, weight, CBC with differential, liver and thyroid function tests, BUN, creatinine, ECG if >40 y.

Drug-Specific Patient Education

• Review target symptoms that drug potentially treats: disruptions in sleep, appetite, concentration, energy, mood; anhedonia; interest; motivation; initiative; suicidal ideation, panic, obsessions, compulsions.

• Review dosing schedule until patient demonstrates a clear understanding of regimen.

• Discuss expected lag period (3–4 wk) before full therapeutic effects can be anticipated.

• Review most common side effects (agitation, anxiety, dizziness, insomnia, nausea, sweating, anorexia, diarrhea, tremor) and encourage patient to report any side effects promptly.

• Educate patient about contraception during drug use.

• Caution patient about concurrent ETOH and drug use.

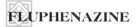

FLUPHENAZINE

Apo-Fluphenazine (CAN),
Moditen Hydrochloride
(CAN), Permitil, Prolixin
  Fluphenazine decanoate

Modecate Decanoate (CAN),
Prolixin Decanoate
  Fluphenazine enanthate

Moditen Enanthate (CAN),
Prolixin Enanthate

PREGNANCY CATEGORY C

Drug Classification: *Type:* dopamine receptor antagonist; also called antipsychotic, neuroleptic, or major tranquilizer; *Class:* phenothiazine; *Subclass:* piperidine.

Mechanisms of Action

Postsynaptic antagonism of dopamine receptors, primarily D2 (antipsychotic efficacy is thought to be mediated by these actions). Blockade of muscarinic cholinergic, noradrenergic, and histaminergic receptors (some undesirable side effects are thought to be mediated by these actions).

Indications

Short- and long-term management of idiopathic psychoses including schizophrenia, schizophreniform disorder, schizoaffective disorder, delusional disorder, brief psychotic disorder, mania with psychosis, and major depressive disorder with psychotic features.

Secondary psychoses associated with a general medical condition or substance-related disorder.

Acute deliria and organic psychoses.

Severe agitation or violent behavior.

Severe behavioral problems in children marked by combativeness and/or explosive hyperexcitability and in the short-term treatment of hyperactive children who show excessive motor activity.

Movement disorder of Huntington's disease.

Motor and vocal tics of Tourette's Syndrome.

Brief use for episodes of severe dyscontrol or apparent psychosis in some personality disorders.

Control of nausea, vomiting, and intractable hiccups.

Contraindications/Cautions

Contraindications: • allergy to fluphenazine • comatose or severely depressed states • presence of large amounts of CNS depressants (alcohol, barbiturates, narcotics, etc.) • bone marrow depression • blood dyscrasias • circulatory collapse • subcortical brain damage • Parkinson's disease • liver damage • cerebral or coronary arteriosclerosis • CV disease • severe hypotension or hypertension • respiratory disorders • glaucoma • history of epilepsy or seizures • peptic ulcer or history of peptic ulcer • decreased renal function • urinary retention, ureteral or urethral spasm • prostate hypertrophy • breast cancer • thyrotoxicosis • myelography within 24 h or scheduled within 48 h • pregnancy • lactation • exposure to heat, organophosphorous insecticides, or atropine or related drugs • children with chickenpox • CNS infections • if signs and symptoms of tardive dyskinesia appear, drug discontinuation should be considered • history of neuroleptic malignant syndrome.

Dosage

Adult: Patients may respond to widely different dosages of antipsychotics. Therefore, there is no set dosage for any given antipsychotic drug. Usual range for acute use (oral): 2–20 mg/d. Usual range for maintenance use (oral): 2–8 mg/d. Can be administered once a day. Decanoate (IM): 12.5 mg to start and 5–50 mg/3 wk maintenance. Enanthate (IM): 12.5 mg to start and 5–75 mg/2 wk. Although controversial, depot forms may be associated with more adverse effects, including tardive dyskinesia, and should probably not be given unless patient is unable to comply with oral medication.

Pediatric Adolescent: Generally not used in children <12 y; >12 y may receive lowest adult dosage.

Geriatric: Start dosage at one-fourth to one-third that given in younger adults and increase more gradually.

Dosage Forms: Tablets: 1, 2.5, 5, 10 mg; Liquid concentrate: 5 mg/ml; Elixir: 0.5 mg/1 ml; Injections (decanoate and enanthate): withdrawal symptoms seen 25 mg/ml.

Pharmacokinetics

Absorption: (oral) adequate but variable; food or antacids may decrease absorption; liquid preparations are absorbed more rapidly and reliably than tablets; onset of action 3–60 min; peak level: 2–4 h; hydrochloride (IM) rapidly and reliably absorbed; onset of action 15–20 min; peak: 30–60 min; decanoate and enanthate (IM) slowly and reliably absorbed; onset of action 24–72 h. *Distribution:* highly protein bound (85–90%) and lipophilic; readily crosses the blood–brain barrier, placenta, and enters breast milk; concentrations in the brain appear to be greater than those in blood; not removed efficiently by dialysis. *Metabolism:* hepatic. *Elimination:* urine. The elimination half-life of most antipsychotic drugs is 18–40 h; plasma levels may vary among individuals by 10- to 20-fold; depot forms (decanoate and enanthate) have elimination half-lives of 3–10 d.

Adverse Effects

CNS: Drowsiness, insomnia, vertigo, headache, weakness, tremors, ataxia, slurring of speech, cerebral edema, seizures, exacerbation of psychotic symptoms, extrapyramidal syndromes (EPS), neuroleptic malignant syndrome, tardive dyskinesia, pseudoparkinsonism, akathisia (see descriptions of symptoms under "Implementation" below).

GI: Dry mouth, salivation, nausea, vomiting, anorexia, constipation, paralytic ileus.

CV: Hypotension, orthostatic hypotension, hypertension, tachycardia, bradycardia, cardiac arrest, CHF, cardiomegaly, refractory arrhythmias, dysrhythmias, pulmonary edema.

RESPIRATORY: Bronchospasm, laryngospasm, dyspnea, suppression of cough reflex, and potential aspiration.

HEMATOLOGIC: Eosinophilia, leukopenia, leukocytosis, anemia, aplastic anemia, hemolytic anemia, thrombocytopenic or nonthrombocytopenic purpura, pancytopenia, elevated serum cholesterol.

GU: Urinary retention, polyuria, incontinence, priapism, ejaculation inhibition, male impotence, urine discolored pink to red-brown.

EENT: Nasal congestion, glaucoma, photophobia, blurred vision, miosis, mydriasis, deposits in the cornea and lens, pigmentary retinopathy.

HYPERSENSITIVITY: Jaundice, urticaria, angioneurotic edema, laryngeal edema, photosensitivity, eczema, asthma, anaphylactoid reactions, exfoliative dermatitis, contact dermatitis.

ENDOCRINE: Lactation, breast engorgement in females, galactorrhea, syndrome of inappropriate ADH secretion, amenorrhea, menstrual irregularities, gynecomastia, changes in libido, hyperglycemia, inhibition of ovulation, infertility, pseudopregnancy, reduced urinary levels of gonadotropins, estrogens, and progestins.

OTHER: Fever, heat stroke, pallor, flushed facies, sweating.

Clinically Important Drug–Drug Interactions

⇥ Additive anticholinergic effects and possibly decreased antipsychotic efficacy with anticholinergic drugs.

⇥ Additive CNS depression and hypotension with barbiturates, alcohol, meperidine.

⇥ Additive effects of both drugs with beta-blockers.

⇥ Increased risk of tachycardia, hypotension with epinephrine, norepinephrine.

⇥ Increased risk of seizure with metrizamide.

⇥ Decreased hypotension effect with guanethidine.

⇥ Because of displacement and competition for protein-binding sites, concomitant treatment with other highly protein-bound medications (e.g., warfarin, digoxin) could alter concentrations of both drugs.

⇥ Decreased effect of oral anticoagulants.

⇥ Possible increase in phenytoin levels.

Lab Test Interference

• False-positive pregnancy tests (less likely if serum test is used).

• Increase in protein-bound iodine not attributable to an increase in thyroxine.

• Blood levels of antipsychotics have not correlated well with clinical response and serum levels are probably more misleading than useful.

Nursing Considerations

Assessment

• Assess for any of the conditions listed under "Contraindications/Cautions" above.

• Assess for alcohol and drug use/abuse and for concomitant use of prescription and/or OTC medications.

• Assess for risk of suicidality.

• Complete physical exam: vital signs including orthostatic BP, ECG, CBC with differential, thyroid and liver function, BUN, creatinine.

Implementation

• Bioavailability differs between brand names of oral forms.

• Dilute liquid concentrate just before administration in 60 ml or more of fruit juice, milk, simple syrup, orange syrup, carbonated beverage, coffee, tea, water, or semisolid foods.

• Protect liquid concentrate from light.

• Give decanoate or enanthate IM injection slowly into upper outer-quadrant of buttock.

• Be alert to potential for aspiration because of suppressed cough reflex.

• Monitor for dehydration, renal or liver abnormalities, depressed WBC, symptoms of infection. Promptly report to prescriber and institute remedial measures.

• Monitor for extrapyramidal side effects (involuntary dystonic muscular movements of the neck, jaw, tongue, or entire body; swallowing difficulties; oculogyric crisis); Parkinsonism (muscle stiffness; cogwheel rigidity; shuffling gait, stooped posture, drooling, coarse tremor, "rabbit syndrome," masklike facies, bradykinesia, akinesia); akathisia (subjective feeling of muscular discomfort that can cause agitation, restlessness, pacing, rocking, continually changing posture, and dysphoria).

• Monitor for symptoms of neuroleptic malignant syndrome: muscle rigidity; altered mental status; evidence of autonomic instability (e.g., irregular pulse or blood pressure, tachycardia, cardiac dysrhythmias); hyperpyrexia, sweating; increased WBC, blood creatinine phosphokinase, liver enzymes, myoglobin; mutism, obtundation, agitation.

• Monitor for symptoms of tardive dyskinesia (abnormal, involuntary, irregular, choreoathetoid movements of muscles of the head, limbs, and trunk; darting, twisting, and protruding movements of the tongue; chewing and lateral jaw movements; lip puckering; facial grimacing; finger movements and hand clenching; torticollis, retrocollis, trunk twisting, pelvic thrusting).

• Taper drug gradually after high-dose therapy due to possible gastritis, nausea, dizziness, headache, tachycardia, insomnia after abrupt withdrawal.

Drug-Specific Patient Education

• Review target symptoms that drug potentially treats: auditory, visual, olfactory, tactile hallucinations; delusions; paranoia; disorders of thought and speech; psychotic agitation; insomnia.

• Review dosing schedule until patient demonstrates a clear

understanding of regimen.
Caution patient against changing dosage or discontinuation
without consulting prescriber.
• Caution patient against concurrent alcohol or drug use.
• Discuss expected lag period
(6 wk or more) before full therapeutic effects appear.
• Review most common side
effects (drowsiness, insomnia,
dry mouth, constipation, dizziness from hypotension, urinary
hesitancy or retention, photosensitivity, blurred vision, urticaria, EPS, Parkinsonism,
akathisia) and encourage patient to report any side effects
promptly.
• If possible, give the patient
full information about the risk
of tardive dyskinesia and possible irreversibility. (The decision
whether to inform patients and/
or their guardians must take
into account the clinical
circumstances and the competency of the patient to understand the information provided.)
• Educate patient about possibly life-threatening blood
dyscrasias and instruct patient
to report fever, chills, sore
throat, unusual bleeding or
bruising, or rash, and to discontinue medication immediately (most likely between 4th
and 10th weeks of treatment).
• Caution patient about risk of
dehydration or heat stroke, increased risk of sunburn, and
warn against over exercising in
a hot climate.

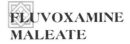

FLUVOXAMINE MALEATE

••••••••••••••••••••••••

Luvox

PREGNANCY CATEGORY C

Drug Classification: *Type:* specific
serotonin reuptake inhibitor
(SSRI); antiobsessive; antidepressant.

Mechanisms of Action
Antiobsessive and antidepressant activity associated with
presynaptic reuptake of serotonin; no significant effects
on norepinephrine,
dopamine.

Indications
Treatment of obsessive-compulsive disorder (OCD), depression, panic disorder, eating disorders

Contraindications/Cautions
Contraindications: • hypersensitivity to fluvoxamine
• MAO inhibitor use • pregnancy • lactation.
  Use cautiously with: • impaired hepatic or renal function • seizures • may cause
mania or hypomania.

Dosage

Adult: 50–3000 mg/d. Given bid. Earliest onset of action within 2–5 d. Consider drug trial a failure if patient has been on maximum recommended dose for 4–6 wk without response.

Pediatric Adolescent: Start at one-half the adult dose and increase slowly and cautiously.

Geriatric: Start at one-half the adult dose and increase slowly and cautiously.

Dosage Forms: Tablets: 50, 100 mg.

Pharmacokinetics

Absorption: from the GI tract; reaches peak plasma levels in 5 h. *Distribution:* 80% protein bound; crosses placenta, enters breast milk. *Metabolism:* hepatic; $T_{1/2}$: 15–16 h. *Steady state:* 7 d; peak plasma levels 3–8 h. *Elimination:* urine.

Adverse Effects

CNS: Headaches, nervousness, insomnia, drowsiness, anxiety, tremor, dizziness, fatigue, asthenia, sedation, sensation disturbance, decreased libido, light-headedness, decreased concentration.

GI: Nausea, diarrhea, dry mouth, anorexia, dyspepsia, constipation, abdominal pain, vomiting, taste change, flatulence, gastroenteritis.

SKIN: Excessive sweating, rash, pruritus.

RESPIRATORY: Flu-like syndrome, pharyngitis, dyspnea, rhinitis.

CV: Hot flashes, palpitations.

GU: Sexual dysfunction, urinary frequency or retention.

Clinically Important Drug–Drug Interactions

⊣ Toxic reactions or serotonin syndrome may occur with MAOIs or L-tryptophan.
⊣ Do not administer with terfenadine, astemizole.
⊣ Increased effects of diazepam, triazolam, midazolam, alprazolam, warfarin, theophylline, carbamazepine, methadone, beta-blockers, diltiazem; reduced dosages of these drugs will be needed.
⊣ Decreased effects of fluvoxamine in cigarette smokers.

Nursing Considerations

Assessment

• Assess for any of the conditions listed in "Contraindications/Cautions" above.
• Assess for concurrent prescription, OTC, or illegal drug or ETOH use/abuse, risk of suicide, and limit drug access to potentially suicidal patients.
• Complete physical, vital signs, weight; CBC with differential; liver and thyroid function tests; BUN; creatinine; ECG if >40 y.

Drug-Specific Patient Education

- Review target symptoms that drug potentially treats: disruptions in sleep, appetite, concentration, energy, mood; anhedonia; interest; motivation; initiative; suicidal ideation, panic, obsessions, compulsions.
- Review dosing schedule until patient demonstrates a clear understanding of regimen.
- Discuss expected lag period (3–4 wk) before full therapeutic effects can be anticipated.
- Review most common side effects (agitation, anxiety, dizziness, insomnia, nausea, sweating, anorexia, diarrhea, tremor) and encourage patient to report any side effects promptly.
- Educate patient about contraception during drug use.
- Caution patient about concurrent ETOH and drug use.

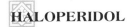

HALOPERIDOL

Haloperidol lactate
   Haloperidol decanoate

Apo-Haloperidol (CAN), Haldol, Haldol Decanoate, Haldol LA (CAN), Novoperidol (CAN), Peridol (CAN)

PREGNANCY CATEGORY C

Drug Classification: *Type:* dopamine receptor antagonist; also called antipsychotic, neuroleptic, or major tranquilizer; *Class:* butyrophenone.

Mechanisms of Action

Postsynaptic antagonism of dopamine receptors, primarily D2 (antipsychotic efficacy is thought to be mediated by these actions). Blockade of muscarinic cholinergic, noradrenergic, and histaminergic receptors (some undesirable side effects are thought to be mediated by these actions).

Indications

Short- and long-term management of idiopathic psychoses including schizophrenia, schizophreniform disorder, schizoaffective disorder, delusional disorder, brief psychotic disorder, mania with psychosis, and major depressive disorder with psychotic features.

Secondary psychoses associated with a general medical condition or substance-related disorder.

Acute deliria and organic psychoses.

Severe agitation or violent behavior.

Severe behavioral problems in children marked by combativeness and/or explosive hyperexcitability and in the short-term treatment of hyperactive children who show excessive motor activity.

Movement disorder of Huntington's disease.

Motor and vocal tics of Tourette's Syndrome.

Brief use for episodes of severe dyscontrol or apparent psychosis in some personality disorders.

Control of nausea, vomiting, and intractable hiccups.

Contraindications/Cautions

Contraindications: • allergy to haloperidol • comatose or severely depressed states • presence of large amounts of CNS depressants (alcohol, barbiturates, narcotics, etc.) • bone marrow depression • blood dyscrasias • circulatory collapse • subcortical brain damage • Parkinson's disease • liver damage • cerebral or coronary arteriosclerosis • CV disease • severe hypotension or hypertension • respiratory disorders • glaucoma • history of epilepsy or seizures • peptic ulcer or history of peptic ulcer • decreased renal function • urinary retention, ureteral or urethral spasm • prostate hypertrophy • breast cancer • thyrotoxicosis • myelography within 24 h or scheduled within 48 h • pregnancy • lactation • exposure to heat, organophosphorous insecticides, or atropine or related drugs • children with chickenpox • CNS infections • if signs and symptoms of tardive dyskinesia appear, drug discontinuation should be considered • history of neuroleptic malignant syndrome.

Dosage

Adult: Patients may respond to widely different dosages of antipsychotics. Therefore, there is no set dosage for any given antipsychotic drug. Usual range for acute use (oral): 2–20 mg/d. Usual range for maintenance use (oral): 1–100 mg/d. Can be administered once a day. IM: oral forms should be used whenever possible, but IM forms may be necessary for patients who exhibit violent behavior or for those who have high first-pass or presystemic metabolism of oral forms. Starting dose of haloperidol lactate: 2–5 mg IM; may repeat in 1 h; increase dosage gradually. Switch to oral dosage as soon as patient is able or willing. Starting dose of decanoate: 75–100 mg q 4 wk (individual dose adjustments will have to be made).

Pediatric Adolescent: Generally not used in children <3 y; 0.5 mg/d PO. May increase 0.5 mg q 5–7 d as needed up to 6 mg/d.

Geriatric: Start dosage at one-fourth to one-third that given in younger adults and increase more gradually.

Dosage Forms: Tablets: 0.5, 1, 2, 5, 10, 20 mg; Liquid concentrate: 2 mg/ml; Injection: lactate 5 mg/ml; decanoate 50 mg/ml, 100 mg/ml.

Pharmacokinetics

Absorption: (oral) adequate but variable; food or antacids may decrease absorption; liquid preparations are absorbed more rapidly and reliably than tablets; onset of action 3–60 min; peak level: 2–4 h; IM rapidly and reliably absorbed; onset of action 15–20 min; peak: 30–60 min. *Distribution:* highly protein bound (85–90%) and lipophilic; readily crosses the blood–brain barrier, placenta, and enters breast milk; concentrations in the brain appear to be greater than those in blood; not removed efficiently by dialysis. *Metabolism:* hepatic. *Elimination:* urine. The elimination half-life of most antipsychotic drugs is 18–40 h; plasma levels may vary among individuals by 10- to 20-fold.

Adverse Effects

CNS: Drowsiness, insomnia, vertigo, headache, weakness, tremors, ataxia, slurring of speech, cerebral edema, seizures, exacerbation of psychotic symptoms, extrapyramidal syndromes (EPS), neuroleptic malignant syndrome, tardive dyskinesia, pseudo-parkinsonism, akathisia (see descriptions of symptoms under "Implementation" below).

GI: Dry mouth, salivation, nausea, vomiting, anorexia, constipation, paralytic ileus.

CV: Hypotension, orthostatic hypotension, hypertension, tachycardia, bradycardia, cardiac arrest, CHF, cardiomegaly, refractory arrhythmias, dysrhythmias, pulmonary edema.

RESPIRATORY: Bronchospasm, laryngospasm, dyspnea, suppression of cough reflex, and potential aspiration.

HEMATOLOGIC: Eosinophilia, leukopenia, leukocytosis, anemia, aplastic anemia, hemolytic anemia, thrombocytopenic or nonthrombocytopenic purpura, pancytopenia, elevated serum cholesterol.

GU: Urinary retention, polyuria, incontinence, priapism, ejaculation inhibition, male impotence, urine discolored pink to red-brown.

EENT: Nasal congestion, glaucoma, photophobia, blurred vision, miosis, mydriasis, deposits in the cornea and lens, pigmentary retinopathy.

HYPERSENSITIVITY: Jaundice, urticaria, angioneurotic edema, laryngeal edema, photosensitivity, eczema, asthma, anaphylactoid reactions, exfoliative dermatitis, contact dermatitis.

ENDOCRINE: Lactation, breast engorgement in females, galactorrhea, syndrome of inappropriate ADH secretion, amenorrhea, menstrual irregularities, gynecomastia, changes in libido, hyperglycemia, inhibition of ovulation, infertility, pseudopregnancy, reduced urinary levels of gonadotropins, estrogens, and progestins.

OTHER: Fever, heat stroke, pallor, flushed facies, sweating.

Clinically Important Drug–Drug Interactions

⇉ Additive anticholinergic effects and possibly decreased antipsychotic efficacy with anticholinergic drugs.
⇉ Additive CNS depression and hypotension with barbiturates, alcohol, meperidine.
⇉ Additive effects of both drugs with beta-blockers.
⇉ Increased risk of tachycardia, hypotension with epinephrine, norepinephrine.
⇉ Increased risk of seizure with metrizamide.
⇉ Decreased hypotension effect with guanethidine.
⇉ Because of displacement and competition for protein-binding sites, concomitant treatment with other highly protein-bound medications (e.g., warfarin, digoxin) could alter concentrations of both drugs.
⇉ Decreased effect of oral anticoagulants.
⇉ Possible increase in phenytoin levels.

Lab Test Interference

• False-positive pregnancy tests (less likely if serum test is used).
• Increase in protein-bound iodine, not attributable to an increase in thyroxine.
• Blood levels of antipsychotics have not correlated well with clinical response and serum levels are probably more misleading than useful.

Nursing Considerations

Assessment
• Assess for any of the conditions listed under "Contraindications/Cautions" above.
• Assess for alcohol and drug use/abuse and for concomitant use of prescription and/or OTC medications.
• Assess for risk of suicidality.
• Complete physical exam: vital signs including orthostatic BP, ECG, CBC with differential, thyroid and liver function, BUN, creatinine.

Implementation
• Bioavailability differs between brand names of oral forms.
• Dilute liquid concentrate just

before administration in 60 ml or more of fruit juice, milk, simple syrup, orange syrup, carbonated beverage, coffee, tea, water, or semisolid foods.
• Protect liquid concentrate from light.
• Give IM injection slowly into upper outer-quadrant of buttock.
• Be alert to potential for aspiration because of suppressed cough reflex.
• Monitor for dehydration, renal or liver abnormalities, depressed WBC, symptoms of infection. Promptly report to prescriber and institute remedial measures.
• Monitor for extrapyramidal side effects (involuntary dystonic muscular movements of the neck, jaw, tongue, or entire body; swallowing difficulties; oculogyric crisis); Parkinsonism (muscle stiffness; cogwheel rigidity; shuffling gait, stooped posture, drooling, coarse tremor, "rabbit syndrome," masklike facies, bradykinesia, akinesia); akathisia (subjective feeling of muscular discomfort that can cause agitation, restlessness, pacing, rocking, continually changing posture, and dysphoria).
• Monitor for symptoms of neuroleptic malignant syndrome: muscle rigidity; altered mental status; evidence of autonomic instability (e.g., irregu-

lar pulse or blood pressure, tachycardia, cardiac dysrhythmias); hyperpyrexia, sweating; increased WBC, blood creatinine phosphokinase, liver enzymes, myoglobin; mutism, obtundation, agitation.
• Monitor for symptoms of tardive dyskinesia (abnormal, involuntary, irregular, choreoathetoid movements of muscles of the head, limbs, and trunk; darting, twisting, and protruding movements of the tongue; chewing and lateral jaw movements; lip puckering; facial grimacing; finger movements and hand clenching; torticollis, retrocollis, trunk twisting, pelvic thrusting).
• Taper drug gradually after high-dose therapy due to possible gastritis, nausea, dizziness, headache, tachycardia, insomnia after abrupt withdrawal.

Drug-Specific Patient Education
• Review target symptoms that drug potentially treats: auditory, visual, olfactory, tactile hallucinations; delusions; paranoia; disorders of thought and speech; psychotic agitation; insomnia.
• Review dosing schedule until patient demonstrates a clear understanding of regimen. Caution patient against changing dosage or discontinuation without consulting prescriber.

• Caution patient against concurrent alcohol or drug use.

• Discuss expected lag period (6 wk or more) before full therapeutic effects appear.

• Review most common side effects (drowsiness, insomnia, dry mouth, constipation, dizziness from hypotension, urinary hesitancy or retention, photosensitivity, blurred vision, urticaria, EPS, Parkinsonism, akathisia) and encourage patient to report any side effects promptly.

• If possible, give the patient full information about the risk of tardive dyskinesia and possible irreversibility. (The decision whether to inform patients and/ or their guardians must take into account the clinical circumstances and the competency of the patient to understand the information provided.)

• Educate patient about possibly life-threatening blood dyscrasias and instruct patient to report fever, chills, sore throat, unusual bleeding or bruising, or rash and to discontinue medication immediately (most likely between 4th and 10th weeks of treatment).

• Caution patient about risk of dehydration or heat stroke, increased risk of sunburn, and warn against over exercising in a hot climate.

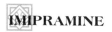

IMIPRAMINE

Imipramine hydrochloride

Apo-Imipramine (CAN), Impril (CAN), Janimine, Novo-pramine (CAN), Tipramine, Tofranil

  Imipramine pamoate

Tofranil-PM

PREGNANCY CATEGORY B

Drug Classification: *Type:* Antidepressant; *Class:* tricyclic (TCA); *Subclass:* tertiary amine.

Mechanisms of Action
Presynaptic reuptake inhibition of neurotransmitters norepinephrine and serotonin (antidepressant efficacy is thought to be mediated by these actions). Postsynaptic blockade of histaminic, muscarinic, and noradrenergic alpha-one and alpha-two receptors (some of the undesirable side effects are thought to be mediated by these actions).

Indications
Relief of symptoms of depression (endogenous depression most responsive).
Enuresis in children 6 y or older.
Unlabeled uses: relief of symptoms of anxiety and panic disorders; control of chronic pain.

Contraindications/Cautions

Contraindications: • hypersensitivity to any tricyclic drug or to tartrazine (in preparations marketed as Janimine, Tofranil, Tofranil-PM; patients with aspirin allergy are often allergic to tartrazine) • concomitant therapy with an MAO inhibitor • ECT with coadministration of TCAs • recent MI • myelography within previous 24 h or scheduled within 48 h.

Use cautiously with: • preexisting CV disorders • seizure disorders • hyperthyroidism • angle-closure glaucoma • increased intraocular pressure • urinary retention • ureteral or urethral spasm • impaired hepatic or renal function • bipolar patients shifting to hypomanic or manic phase • elective surgery • pregnancy • lactation.

Dosage

Adult: Typical starting dose 50 mg qhs. Can be administered once a day, usually at hs, or in divided doses if patient has side effects due to high peak levels. Increase by 50 mg q 3–4 d as side effects allow. Usual maintenance dose 150–200 mg/d. Extreme dose 300 mg qd. Earliest onset of action 2–5 d. Consider drug trial a failure if patient has been on maximal dose for 4–6 wk without response. Limit potentially suicidal patients' access to drug. IM may only be given to patients unable or unwilling to take PO; up to 100 mg/d in divided doses. Replace with PO as soon as possible. Panic disorder: may be necessary to start as low as 10 mg/d.

Pediatric Adolescent: 40 mg/d; doses >100 mg/d generally are not needed.

Childhood enuresis (6 y or older): Initially 25 mg/d 1 h before bedtime. If response is not satisfactory after 1 wk, increase to 50 mg nightly in children <12 y; 75 mg/d does not have greater efficacy but is more likely to increase side effects. Do not exceed 2.5 mg/kg per day. Early night bed wetters may be more effectively treated with earlier and divided dosage (25 mg midafternoon, repeated hs). Institute drug-free period after successful therapy, gradually tapering dosage.

Geriatric: Initially 10 mg/d. Adjust dose according to tolerance and blood level.

Dosage Forms: Tablets: 10, 25, 50, 75, 100, 125, 150 mg; ampules IM: 25 mg/2 ml.

Blood Levels: Draw only to assess compliance; to confirm rapid or slow metabolizers; to document adequate drug trial. Patients with a combined level of imipramine/desipramine greater than 225 ng/ml may improve more than those below that level. Levels should be drawn when any dose has reached steady state (5–7 d) and 10–14 h after last dose.

Pharmacokinetics

Absorption: from GI tract rapidly and completely. *Distribution:* highly lipophilic and largely protein bound; crosses blood–brain barrier and placenta and enters breast milk. *Metabolism:* hepatic; $T_{1/2}$: 48–72 h. *Elimination:* urine. *Peak level:* 2–4 h. *Steady state:* 5 d.

Adverse Effects

Adult Use

CNS: *Sedation and anticholinergic effects*—dry mouth, blurred vision, disturbance of accommodation for near vision, mydriasis, increased intraocular pressure; confusion, disturbed concentration, hallucinations, disorientation, decreased memory, feelings of unreality, delusions, anxiety, nervousness, restlessness, agitation, panic, insomnia, nightmares, hypomania, mania, exacerbation of psychosis, drowsiness, weakness, fatigue, headache, numbness, tingling, paresthesias of extremities, discoordination, motor hyperactivity, akathisia, ataxia, tremors, peripheral neuropathy, extrapyramidal symptoms, seizures, speech blockage, dysarthria, tinnitus, altered EEG.

GI: Dry mouth, constipation, paralytic ileus, nausea, vomiting, anorexia, epigastric distress, diarrhea, flatulence, dysphagia, peculiar taste, increased salivation, stomatitis, glossitis, parotid swelling, abdominal cramps, black tongue, hepatitis.

CV: Orthostatic hypotension, hypertension, syncope, tachycardia, palpitations, MI, arrhythmias, heart block, precipitation of CHF, stroke.

HEMATOLOGIC: Bone marrow depression, including agranulocytosis; eosinophilia, purpura, thrombocytopenia, leukopenia.

GU: Urinary retention, delayed micturition, dilation of the urinary tract, gynecomastia, testicular swelling in men; breast enlargement, menstrual irregularity, and galactorrhea in women; increased or decreased libido; impotence.

HYPERSENSITIVITY: Skin rash, pruritus, vasculitis, petechiae, photosensitization, edema (generalized, facial, tongue), drug fever.

ENDOCRINE: Elevated or depressed blood sugar, elevated prolactin levels, inappropriate ADH secretion.

WITHDRAWAL: Abrupt discontinuation of prolonged

therapy: nausea, headache, vertigo, nightmares, malaise.

OTHER: Nasal congestion, excessive appetite, weight gain or loss; sweating (paradoxical effect in a drug with prominent anticholinergic effects), alopecia, lacrimation, hyperthermia, flushing, chills.

Pediatric Use for Enuresis

CNS: Nervousness, sleep disorders, tiredness, convulsions, anxiety, emotional instability, syncope, collapse.

GI: Constipation, mild GI disturbances.

CV: ECG changes of unknown significance when given in doses of 5 mg/kg per day.

OTHER: Adverse effects reported with adult use.

Clinically Important Drug–Drug Interactions

⌗ Increased sedation with alcohol, antihistamines, antipsychotics, barbiturates, chloral hydrate, and other sedatives.
⌗ Increased hypotension with alpha-methyldopa, beta-adrenergic blockers, clonidine, diuretics, low-potency antipsychotics.
⌗ Additive cardiotoxicity with quinidine and other class II antiarrhythmics, thioridazine, mesoridazine, pimozide.
⌗ Additive anticholinergic toxicity with antihistamines, antiparkinsonians, low-potency antipsychotics, especially thioridazine, over-the-counter sleeping medications, gastrointestinal antispasmodics and antidiarrheals.
⌗ TCAs may increase the effects of warfarin and block the effects of guanethidine.
⌗ Increased sympathomimetic (especially alpha-adrenergic) effects of direct-acting sympathomimetic drugs (norepinephrine, epinephrine).
⌗ Decreased effects of indirect-acting sympathomimetic drugs (ephedrine).
⌗ Increased levels and possible delirium with disulfiram.

Note: MAOIs and TCAs have been used successfully in some patients who are resistant to therapy with single agents; however, hyperpyretic crises, severe convulsions, hypertensive episodes, and deaths can occur when MAOIs are given with TCAs.

Nursing Considerations

Assessment

• Assess for any of the conditions listed under "Contraindications/Cautions" above.
• Assess for ETOH and drug use/abuse and for prescription and/or OTC medications.
• Assess for suicidal ideation

• Complete physical exam: vital signs, EKG for patients 40 y or older, CBC with differential, thyroid function, liver function, BUN, creatinine, weight changes, I & O, vision; sexual interest, function, and activity.

Drug-Specific Patient Education
• Review target symptoms that drug potentially treats: disruptions in sleep, appetite, concentration, energy, mood; anhedonia; interest; motivation; initiative.
• Review dosing schedule until patient demonstrates a clear understanding of regimen.
• Discuss expected lag period (3–4 wk) before therapeutic effects can be anticipated.
• Review most common side effects: dry mouth, constipation, dizziness, urinary hesitancy, headache, nausea, sedation, or agitation, and encourage patient to report any side effects promptly.
• Caution patient against abrupt discontinuation without consulting prescriber. Abrupt discontinuation may cause withdrawal symptoms (cholinergic rebound, malaise, chills, coryza, muscle aches, agitation, insomnia) or rapid reemergence of depressive symptoms.
• Caution patient about ETOH and drug use.

LITHIUM

Lithium carbonate

Carbolith (CAN), Duralith (CAN), Eskalith, Lithane, Lithizine (CAN), Lithonate, Lithotabs

Lithium citrate

Cibalith-S

PREGNANCY CATEGORY D

Drug Classification: *Type:* antimanic agent; *Class:* metal.

Mechanisms of Action
Mechanism of action is not completely known; alters sodium transport in nerve and muscle cells. Inhibits release of norepinephrine and dopamine, but not serotonin, from stimulated neurons. Slightly increases intraneuronal stores of catecholamines. Decreases intraneuronal content of second messengers and may, thereby, selectively modulate the responsiveness of hyperactive neurons that might contribute to the manic state.

Indications
Treatment of manic episodes of manic-depressive illness.
Maintenance therapy to prevent or diminish the frequency and intensity of subsequent manic episodes

Contraindications/Cautions

Contraindications: • hypersensitivity to tartrazine (in tablets marketed as *Lithane*) • significant renal or cardiovascular disease • severe debilitation, dehydration • sodium depletion, patients on diuretics • pregnancy • lactation.

Use cautiously with: sweating, diarrhea • suicidal or impulsive patients • infection with fever.

Dosage

Individualize dosage according to serum levels and clinical response.

Adult: *Acute mania:* 600 mg PO tid or 900 mg slow release form PO bid, to produce effective serum levels between 1 and 1.5 mEq/L. Serum levels should be determined twice weekly in samples drawn immediately before a dose and 8–12 h after the previous dose.

Long-term use: 300 mg PO tid–qid, to produce a serum level of 0.6–1.2 mEq/L. Serum levels should be determined at least every 2 mo in samples drawn immediately before a dose and 8–12 h after the previous dose. *Conversion from conventional to slow release dosage forms:* Give same total daily dose divided into 2 or 3 doses.

Pediatric: Safety and efficacy for children under 12 y not established.

Geriatric and Renal Impaired: Reduced dosage may be necessary. Elderly patients often respond to reduced dosage and may exhibit signs of toxicity at serum levels tolerated by other patients. Plasma half-life is prolonged in renal impairment.

Dosage Forms: Capsules: 150, 300, 600 mg; Controlled release tablets: 450 mg; Syrup: 300 mg/5 ml.

Blood Levels: 0.8–1.5 mEq/L.

Pharmacokinetics

Absorption: rapidly from the GI tract. *Distribution:* not protein-bound; crosses placenta and enters breast milk. *Metabolism:* not metabolized. *Onset:* 5–14 d. *Steady state:* 10–21 d. *Elimination:* urine.

Adverse Effects

Reactions are related to serum lithium levels (toxic lithium levels are close to therapeutic levels): therapeutic levels in acute mania range between 1 and 1.5 mEq/L; therapeutic levels for maintenance are 0.6–1.2 mEq/L).

<1.5 mEq/L

GI: Nausea, vomiting, diarrhea, thirst.

GU: Polyuria.

CNS: Lethargy, slurred

speech, muscle weakness, fine hand-tremor.

1.5–2.0 mEq/L (mild to moderate toxic reactions)

GI: Persistent GI upset, gastritis, salivary gland swelling, abdominal pain, excessive salivation, flatulence, indigestion.

CNS: Coarse hand tremor, mental confusion, hyperirritability of muscles, drowsiness, incoordination.

CV: ECG changes.

2.0–2.5 mEq/L (moderate to severe toxic reactions)

CNS: Ataxia, giddiness, fasciculations, tinnitus, blurred vision, clonic movements, seizures, stupor, coma.

CV: Serious ECG changes, severe hypotension.

GU: Large output of dilute urine.

RESPIRATORY: Fatalities secondary to pulmonary complications.

>2.5 mEq/L (*life-threatening toxicity*)

GENERAL: Complex involvement of multiple organ systems.

Reactions unrelated to serum levels

CNS: Headache, worsening of organic brain syndromes, fever, reversible short-term memory impairment, dyspraxia.

CV: ECG changes; hyperkalemia associated with ECG changes; syncope; tachybradycardia syndrome; rarely, arrhythmias, CHF, diffuse myocarditis, death.

GI: Dysgeusia/taste distortion, salty taste; swollen lips; dental caries.

DERMATOLOGIC: Pruritus with or without rash; maculopapular, acneiform and follicular eruptions; cutaneous ulcers; edema of ankles or wrists.

ENDOCRINE: Diffuse nontoxic goiter; hypercalcemia-associated with hyperparathyroidism; transient hyperglycemia; irreversible nephrogenic diabetes insipidus that improves with diuretic therapy; impotence/sexual dysfunction.

MISCELLANEOUS: Weight gain (5–10 kg); chest tightness; reversible respiratory failure; swollen and/or painful joints, eye irritation, worsening of cataracts, disturbance of visual accommodation.

Clinically Important Drug–Drug Interactions

⇥ Increased risk of toxicity when given with thiazide diuretics due to decreased renal clearance of lithium.

⇥ Increased plasma lithium levels with indomethacin, some other NSAIDs—phenylbutazone, piroxicam, ibuprofen.

⇥ Increased CNS toxicity of lithium when given with carbamazepine.

⇥ Encephalopathic syndrome

(weakness, lethargy, fever, tremulousness, confusion, extrapyramidal symptoms, leucocytosis, elevated serum enzymes) with irreversible brain damage when taken with haloperidol.

⧫ Greater risk of hypothyroidism when given with iodide salts.

⧫ Decreased effectiveness of lithium, due to increased excretion of lithium, when given with urinary alkalinizers, including antacids, tromethamine.

Nursing Considerations

Assessment

• Assess for any conditions listed under "Contraindications/Cautions" above.

• Assess for history or alcohol or drug abuse or dependence, use of current prescribed or OTC medications.

• Complete physical exam: vital signs, thyroid and renal glomerular and tubular function tests, urinalysis, CBC and differential.

• Assess for adequate daily intake of salt and fluid (2500–3000 ml/d).

• Assess serum lithium levels periodically, daily with severe renal or cardiovascular diseases, debilitation, dehydration.

Drug-Specific Patient Education

• Review the target symptoms that the drug potentially treats: signs of mania.

• Review the dosing schedule until patient demonstrates a clear understanding of drug regimen, including taking drug after meals or with food or milk.

• Review the most common side effects: drowsiness, dizziness; GI upset; mild thirst; greater than usual urine volume; fine hand-tremor.

• Review the side effects patient should report promptly: diarrhea, vomiting, ataxia, tremor, drowsiness, lack of coordination or muscular weakness, fever, diarrhea.

• Caution patient to eat a normal diet with normal salt intake; maintain adequate fluid intake (at least 2½ quarts/d).

• Caution patient to keep appointments for regular blood tests while on this drug.

• Caution patient to avoid pregnancy, use of a barrier contraceptive is advised.

• Caution patient to avoid alcohol and sleep-inducing or OTC medications.

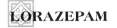

LORAZEPAM

Apo-Lorazepam (CAN), Ativan, Novolorazem (CAN)

PREGNANCY CATEGORY D

C-IV controlled substance

Drug Classification: *Type:* anxiolytic; *Class:* 3-hydroxy-benzodiazepine

Mechanisms of Action

Benzodiazepines bind to specific receptor sites associated with the major inhibitory neurotransmitter in the brain, gamma-aminobutyric acid (GABA), thereby increasing the affinity of the receptor sites. While the exact mechanisms of action are not completely understood, inhibitory actions on neurons within the limbic system, and on serotonergic (5-HT) and noradrenergic neurons within the brainstem, are responsible for the anxiolytic properties.

Indications

Relief of symptoms of anxiety.
Symptomatic relief of acute alcohol withdrawal.
Management of psychotic agitation.
Treatment of akathisia.
Management of status epilepticus.

Contraindications/Cautions

Contraindications: • hypersensitivity to benzodiazepines • psychoses, acute narrow-angle glaucoma, shock, coma, acute alcoholic intoxication • pregnancy (cleft lip or palate, inguinal hernia, cardiac defects, microcephaly, pyloric stenosis when used in first trimester; neonatal withdrawal syndrome reported in babies) • lactation.
   Use cautiously with: • patients with history of alcohol or drug dependence or addiction • elderly or debilitated patients • patients with impaired liver or kidney function.

Dosage

Adult: 30–120 mg/d; may be given bid–qid.

Pediatric Adolescent: <12 y dosage not established.

Geriatric: Initial dose 10 mg/d; adjust dose according to tolerance and remission of symptoms.

Dosage Forms: Tablets: 15 mg; Capsules: 10, 15, 30 mg.

Pharmacokinetics

Absorption: from GI tract at slow rate with rapid onset of action. *Distribution:* highly lipid soluble, crosses placenta, passes into breast milk. *Metabolism:* hepatic; $T_{1/2}$: 10–30 h. *Peak plasma level:* 2–4 h. *Steady state:* up to 1 wk. *Elimination:* urine.

Adverse Effects

CNS: Transient, mild drowsiness initially; sedation, fatigue, ataxia; confusion, depression, lethargy, stupor, apathy, lightheadedness, disorientation, dysarthria, headache, slurred speech, tremor, vertigo, diplopia, nystagmus, paradoxical excitatory reactions, anxiety, hallucinations, euphoria, difficulty in concentration, vivid dreams, psychomotor retardation increased muscle spasticity, insomnia, rage, sleep disturbances, minor changes in EEG patterns.

GI: Constipation, changes in salivation, nausea, anorexia, vomiting, difficulty in swallowing, elevations of blood enzymes—LDH, alkaline phosphatase, SGOT, SGPT; hepatic dysfunction, jaundice.

CV: Bradycardia, tachycardia, hypertension and hypotension, palpitations, edema.

HEMATOLOGIC: Neutropenia, blood dyscrasias.

GU: Incontinence, urinary retention, changes in libido.

DERMATOLOGIC: Skin rashes.

TOLERANCE/DEPENDENCE: Some patients report a tolerance to the anxiolytic effects of benzodiazepines and require increased doses to maintain clinical remission. There is also a cross-tolerance among most of the benzodiazepines. Abrupt discontinuation, particularly of those with short half-lives, is associated with severe withdrawal symptoms seen only in patients who have taken high doses for long periods. Appearance of the syndrome may be delayed for 1–2 wk with benzodiazepines with very long half-lives. Commonly observed withdrawal symptoms in benzodiazepine withdrawal syndrome: anxiety, irritability, insomnia, fatigue, headache, muscle twitching or aching, tremor, shakiness, sweating, dizziness, concentration difficulties, nausea, anorexia, observable depression, depersonalization, derealization, increased sensory perception, abnormal perception or sensation of movement.

Clinically Important Drug–Drug Interactions

- Decreased absorption with antacids.
- Increased CNS depression with antihistamines, barbiturates and similarly acting drugs, cyclic antidepressants, alcohol, omeprazole.
- Increased benzodiazepine level with cimetidine, disulfiram, erythromycin, estrogens, fluoxetine, isoniazid.
- Decreased benzodiazepine levels with carbamazepine and, possibly, other anticonvulsants, theophyllines, ranitidine.

Nursing Considerations

Assessment

- Assess for any of the conditions listed under "Contraindications/Cautions" above.
- Assess for current use or history of alcohol or drug depen-

dence or abuse, use of concurrent prescribed or OTC medications.
• Patient should have had routine complete physical within last year.
• Monitor vital signs during acute alcohol withdrawal; liver and kidney function; CBC with differential during long-term therapy.
• If discontinuing, taper dosage gradually (25% per week) and monitor for withdrawal symptoms.

Drug-Specific Patient Education
• Review symptoms specific to individual patient which drug potentially treats (anxiety, alcohol withdrawal, panic, phobias, insomnia).
• Review dosing schedule until patient demonstrates a clear understanding of regimen.
• Discuss expected onset of action.
• Review most common side effects (drowsiness, fatigue, ataxia) and encourage patient to report any side effects promptly.
• Caution patient about possible tolerance and/or psychological and physical dependence.
• Warn against abrupt discontinuation.
• Review possible withdrawal symptoms (see above under "Tolerance/Dependence").

LOXAPINE

Loxapine hydrochloride

Loxitane-C, Loxitane
    Loxapine succinate

Loxapac (CAN), Loxitane

PREGNANCY CATEGORY C

Drug Classification: *Type:* dopamine receptor antagonist; also called antipsychotic, neuroleptic, or major tranquilizer; *Class:* dibenzoxazepine; *Subclass:* piperazine.

Mechanisms of Action
Postsynaptic antagonism of dopamine receptors, primarily D2 (antipsychotic efficacy is thought to be mediated by these actions). Blockade of muscarinic cholinergic, noradrenergic, and histaminergic receptors (some undesirable side effects are thought to be mediated by these actions).

Indications
Short- and long-term management of idiopathic psychoses including schizophrenia, schizophreniform disorder, schizoaffective disorder, delusional disorder, brief psychotic disorder, mania with psychosis, and major depressive disorder with psychotic features.

Secondary psychoses associated with a general medical condition or substance-related disorder.

Acute deliria and organic psychoses.

Severe agitation or violent behavior.

Severe behavioral problems in children marked by combativeness and/or explosive hyperexcitability, and in the short-term treatment of hyperactive children who show excessive motor activity.

Movement disorder of Huntington's disease.

Motor and vocal tics of Tourette's Syndrome.

Brief use for episodes of severe dyscontrol or apparent psychosis in some personality disorders.

Control of nausea, vomiting, and intractable hiccups.

Contraindications/Cautions

Contraindications: • allergy to loxapine • comatose or severely depressed states • presence of large amounts of CNS depressants (alcohol, barbiturates, narcotics, etc.) • bone marrow depression • blood dyscrasias • circulatory collapse • subcortical brain damage • Parkinson's disease • liver damage • cerebral or coronary arteriosclerosis • CV disease • severe hypotension or hypertension • respiratory disorders • glaucoma • history of epilepsy or seizures • peptic ulcer or history of peptic ulcer • decreased renal function • urinary retention, ureteral or urethral spasm • prostate hypertrophy • breast cancer • thyrotoxicosis • myelography within 24 h or scheduled within 48 h • pregnancy • lactation • exposure to heat, organophosphorous insecticides, or atropine or related drugs • children with chickenpox • CNS infections • if signs and symptoms of tardive dyskinesia appear, drug discontinuation should be considered • history of neuroleptic malignant syndrome

Dosage

Adult: Patients may respond to widely different dosages of antipsychotics. Therefore, there is no set dosage for any given antipsychotic drug. Usual range for acute use (oral): 50–250 mg/d. Usual range for maintenance use (oral): 20–100 mg/d. Can be administered once a day. IM: oral forms should be used whenever possible, but IM forms may be necessary for patients who exhibit violent behavior or for those who have high first-pass or presystemic metabolism of oral forms. Starting dose 50 mg IM; may repeat in 1 h; increase dosage gradually up to 50 mg q 4–6 h. Switch to oral dosage as soon as patient is able or willing.

Pediatric Adolescent: Generally not used in children <16 y; >16 y give lowest adult dosage.

Geriatric: Start dosage at one-fourth to one-third that given in younger adults and increase more gradually.

Dosage Forms: Tablets: 5, 10, 25, 50 mg; Liquid concentrate: 25 mg/ml; Injection: 50 mg/ml.

Pharmacokinetics

Absorption: (oral) adequate but variable; food or antacids may decrease absorption; liquid preparations are absorbed more rapidly and reliably than tablets; onset of action 3–60 min; peak level: 2–4 h; IM rapidly and reliably absorbed; onset of action 15–20 min; peak: 30–60 min. *Distribution:* highly protein bound (85–90%) and lipophilic; readily crosses the blood–brain barrier, placenta and enters breast milk; concentrations in the brain appear to be greater than those in blood; not removed efficiently by dialysis. *Metabolism:* hepatic. *Elimination:* urine. The elimination half-life of most antipsychotic drugs is 18–40 h; plasma levels may vary among individuals by 10- to 20-fold.

Adverse Effects

CNS: Drowsiness, insomnia, vertigo, headache, weakness, tremors, ataxia, slurring of speech, cerebral edema, seizures, exacerbation of psychotic symptoms, extrapyramidal syndromes (EPS), neuroleptic malignant syndrome, tardive dyskinesia, pseudo-parkinsonism, akathisia (see descriptions of symptoms under "Implementation" below).

GI: Dry mouth, salivation, nausea, vomiting, anorexia, constipation, paralytic ileus.

CV: Hypotension, orthostatic hypotension, hypertension, tachycardia, bradycardia, cardiac arrest, CHF, cardiomegaly, refractory arrhythmias, dysrhythmias, pulmonary edema.

RESPIRATORY: Bronchospasm, laryngospasm, dyspnea, suppression of cough reflex, and potential aspiration.

HEMATOLOGIC: Eosinophilia, leukopenia, leukocytosis, anemia, aplastic anemia, hemolytic anemia, thrombocytopenic or nonthrombocytopenic purpura, pancytopenia, elevated serum cholesterol.

GU: Urinary retention, polyuria, incontinence, priapism, ejaculation inhibition, male impotence, urine discolored pink to red-brown.

EENT: Nasal congestion, glaucoma, photophobia, blurred vision, miosis, mydriasis, deposits in the cornea and lens, pigmentary retinopathy.

HYPERSENSITIVITY: Jaundice, urticaria, angioneurotic edema, laryngeal edema, photosensitivity, eczema, asthma, anaphylactoid reactions, exfoliative dermatitis, contact dermatitis.

ENDOCRINE: Lactation, breast engorgement in females, galactorrhea, syndrome of inappropriate ADH secretion, amenorrhea, menstrual irregularities, gynecomastia, changes in libido, hyperglycemia, inhibition of ovulation, infertility, pseudopregnancy, reduced urinary levels of gonadotropins, estrogens, and progestins.

OTHER: Fever, heat stroke, pallor, flushed facies, sweating.

Clinically Important Drug–Drug Interactions

⊬ Additive anticholinergic effects and possibly decreased antipsychotic efficacy with anticholinergic drugs.
⊬ Additive CNS depression and hypotension with barbiturates, alcohol, meperidine.
⊬ Additive effects of both drugs with beta-blockers.
⊬ Increased risk of tachycardia, hypotension with epinephrine, norepinephrine.

⊬ Increased risk of seizure with metrizamide.
⊬ Decreased hypotension effect with guanethidine.
⊬ Because of displacement and competition for protein-binding sites, concomitant treatment with other highly protein-bound medications (e.g., warfarin, digoxin) could alter concentrations of both drugs.
⊬ Decreased effect of oral anticoagulants.
⊬ Possible increase in phenytoin levels.

Lab Test Interference

• False-positive pregnancy tests (less likely if serum test is used).
• Increase in protein-bound iodine, not attributable to an increase in thyroxine.
• Blood levels of antipsychotics have not correlated well with clinical response and serum levels are probably more misleading than useful.

Nursing Considerations

Assessment

• Assess for any of the conditions listed under "Contraindications/Cautions" above.
• Assess for alcohol and drug use/abuse and for concomitant use of prescription and/or OTC medications.
• Assess for risk of suicidality.
• Complete physical exam: vital signs including orthostatic BP, ECG, CBC with differential,

thyroid and liver function, BUN, creatinine.

Implementation
• Bioavailability differs between brand names of oral forms.
• Dilute liquid concentrate just before administration in 60 ml or more of fruit juice, milk, simple syrup, orange syrup, carbonated beverage, coffee, tea, water, or semisolid foods.
• Protect liquid concentrate from light.
• Give IM injection slowly into upper outer-quadrant of buttock.
• Be alert to potential for aspiration because of suppressed cough reflex.
• Monitor for dehydration, renal or liver abnormalities, depressed WBC, symptoms of infection. Promptly report to prescriber and institute remedial measures.
• Monitor for extrapyramidal side effects (involuntary dystonic muscular movements of the neck, jaw, tongue, or entire body; swallowing difficulties; oculogyric crisis); Parkinsonism (muscle stiffness; cogwheel rigidity; shuffling gait, stooped posture, drooling, coarse tremor, "rabbit syndrome," masklike facies, bradykinesia, akinesia); akathisia (subjective feeling of muscular discomfort that can cause agitation, restlessness, pacing, rocking, continually changing posture, and dysphoria).

• Monitor for symptoms of neuroleptic malignant syndrome: muscle rigidity; altered mental status; evidence of autonomic instability (e.g., irregular pulse or blood pressure, tachycardia, cardiac dysrhythmias); hyperpyrexia, sweating; increased WBC, blood creatinine phosphokinase, liver enzymes, myoglobin; mutism, obtundation, agitation.
• Monitor for symptoms of tardive dyskinesia (abnormal, involuntary, irregular, choreoathetoid movements of muscles of the head, limbs, and trunk; darting, twisting, and protruding movements of the tongue; chewing and lateral jaw movements; lip puckering; facial grimacing; finger movements and hand clenching; torticollis, retrocollis, trunk twisting, pelvic thrusting).
• Taper drug gradually after high-dose therapy due to possible gastritis, nausea, dizziness, headache, tachycardia, insomnia after abrupt withdrawal.

Drug-Specific Patient Education
• Review target symptoms that drug potentially treats: auditory, visual, olfactory, tactile hallucinations; delusions; paranoia; disorders of thought and speech; psychotic agitation; insomnia.
• Review dosing schedule until patient demonstrates a clear

understanding of regimen. Caution patient against changing dosage or discontinuation without consulting prescriber.

• Caution patient against concurrent alcohol or drug use.

• Discuss expected lag period (6 wk or more) before full therapeutic effects appear.

• Review most common side effects (drowsiness, insomnia, dry mouth, constipation, dizziness from hypotension, urinary hesitancy or retention, photosensitivity, blurred vision, urticaria, EPS, Parkinsonism, akathisia) and encourage patient to report any side effects promptly.

• If possible, give the patient full information about the risk of tardive dyskinesia and possible irreversibility. (The decision whether to inform patients and/or their guardians must take into account the clinical circumstances and the competency of the patient to understand the information provided.)

• Educate patient about possibly life-threatening blood dyscrasias and instruct patient to report fever, chills, sore throat, unusual bleeding or bruising, or rash and to discontinue medication immediately (most likely between 4th and 10th weeks of treatment).

• Caution patient about risk of dehydration or heat stroke, increased risk of sunburn, and warn against over exercising in a hot climate.

MAPROTILINE HYDROCHLORIDE

Ludiomil

PREGNANCY CATEGORY C

Drug Classification: *Type:* Antidepressant; *Class:* tetracyclic; *Subclass:* secondary amine.

Mechanisms of Action

Presynaptic reuptake inhibition of neurotransmitters norepinephrine (primarily) and serotonin (antidepressant efficacy is thought to be mediated by these actions). Postsynaptic blockade of histaminic, muscarinic, and noradrenergic alpha-one and alpha-two receptors (some of the undesirable side effects are thought to be mediated by these actions).

Indications

Relief of symptoms of depression (endogenous depression most responsive).

Contraindications/Cautions

Contraindications: • hypersensitivity to any tricyclic drug • concomitant therapy with an MAO inhibitor • ECT with coadministration of TCAs • recent MI • myelography within previous 24 h or scheduled within 48 h.

Use cautiously with: • preexisting CV disorders, especially cardiac conduction system disease • seizure disorders • hyperthyroidism • angle-closure glaucoma • increased intraocular pressure • urinary retention • ureteral or urethral spasm • impaired hepatic or renal function • bipolar patients shifting to hypomanic or manic phase • elective surgery • pregnancy • lactation.

Dosage

Adult: Typical starting dose 25 mg qhs. Can be administered once a day, usually at hs. Divided doses if patient has side effects due to high peak levels. Increase by 25 mg q 3–4 d as side effects allow. Usual maintenance dose 150–225 mg/d. Earliest onset of action in 2–5 d. Consider drug trial a failure if patient has been on maximal dose for 4–6 wk without response. Limit potentially suicidal patients' access to drug.

Pediatric Adolescent: Not recommended in children <18 y.

Geriatric: Initially 25 mg/d. Adjust dose according to tolerance and blood level.

Dosage Forms: Tablets: 25, 50, 75 mg.

Blood Levels: Draw only to assess compliance; to confirm rapid or slow metabolizers; to document adequate drug trial. Therapeutic range is 50–300 ng/ml; greater than 150 ng/ml may reduce efficacy; levels should be drawn when any dose has reached steady state (5–7 d) and 10–14 h after last dose.

Pharmacokinetics

Absorption: from GI tract rapidly and completely. *Distribution:* highly lipophilic and largely protein bound; crosses blood–brain barrier and placenta and enters breast milk. *Metabolism:* hepatic; $T_{1/2}$: 43–51 h. *Elimination:* urine and feces. *Steady state:* 5–7 d.

Adverse Effects

Adult Use

CNS: Sedation and anticholinergic effects—dry mouth, blurred vision, disturbance of accommodation for near vision, mydriasis, increased intraocular pressure; confusion, disturbed concentration, hallucinations, disorientation, decreased memory, feelings of unreality, delusions, anxiety, nervousness, restlessness, agitation, panic, insomnia, nightmares, hypomania, mania, exacerbation of psychosis, drowsiness, weakness, fatigue, headache, numbness, tingling, paresthesias of extremities, discoordination, motor hyperactivity, akathisia, ataxia, tremors, peripheral neuropathy, extrapyramidal symptoms, seizures, speech blockage, dysarthria, tinnitus, altered EEG.

GI: Dry mouth, constipation, paralytic ileus, nausea, vomiting, anorexia, epigastric distress, diarrhea, flatulence, dysphagia, peculiar taste, increased salivation, stomatitis, glossitis, parotid swelling, abdominal cramps, black tongue, hepatitis.

CV: Orthostatic hypotension, hypertension, syncope, tachycardia, palpitations, MI, arrhythmias, heart block, precipitation of CHF, stroke.

HEMATOLOGIC: Bone marrow depression, including agranulocytosis; eosinophilia, purpura, thrombocytopenia.

GU: Urinary retention, delayed micturition, dilation of the urinary tract, gynecomastia, testicular swelling in men; breast enlargement, menstrual irregularity and galactorrhea in women; increased or decreased libido; impotence.

HYPERSENSITIVITY: Skin rash, pruritus, vasculitis, petechiae, photosensitization, edema (generalized, facial, tongue), drug fever.

ENDOCRINE: Elevated or depressed blood sugar, elevated prolactin levels, inappropriate ADH secretion.

WITHDRAWAL: Abrupt discontinuation of prolonged therapy: nausea, headache, vertigo, nightmares, malaise.

OTHER: Nasal congestion, excessive appetite, weight gain or loss; sweating (paradoxical effect in a drug with prominent anticholinergic effects), alopecia, lacrimation, hyperthermia, flushing, chills.

Clinically Important Drug–Drug Interactions

⧧ Increased sedation with alcohol, antihistamines, antipsychotics, barbiturates, chloral hydrate, and other sedatives.

⧧ Increased hypotension with alpha-methyldopa, beta-adrenergic blockers, clonidine, diuretics, low-potency antipsychotics.

⧧ Additive cardiotoxicity with quinidine and other class II antiarrhythmics, thioridazine, mesoridazine, pimozide.

⧧ Additive anticholinergic toxicity with antihistamines, antiparkinsonians, low-potency antipsychotics, especially thioridazine, over-the-counter sleeping medications, gastrointestinal antispasmodics and antidiarrheals.

⧧ TCAs may increase the effects of warfarin and block the effects of guanethidine.

⧧ Increased sympathomimetic (especially alpha-adrenergic) effects of direct acting sympathomimetic drugs (norepinephrine, epinephrine).

⧧ Decreased effects of indirect-acting sympathomimetic drugs (ephedrine).

⊬ Increased levels and possible delirium with disulfiram.

Note: MAOIs and TCAs have been used successfully in some patients who are resistant to therapy with single agents; however, hyperpyretic crises, severe convulsions, hypertensive episodes, and deaths can occur when MAOIs are given with TCAs.

Nursing Considerations

Assessment
• Assess for any of the conditions listed under "Contraindications/Cautions" above.
• Assess for ETOH or drug use/abuse and for concomitant prescribed and/or OTC medications.
• Complete physical exam: vital signs, EKG for patients 40 y or older, CBC with differential, thyroid function, liver function, BUN, creatinine, weight changes, I & O, vision; sexual interest, function, and activity.

Drug-Specific Patient Education
• Review target symptoms that drug potentially treats: disruptions in sleep, appetite concentration, energy, mood; anhedonia; interest; motivation; initiative.
• Review dosing schedule until patient demonstrates a clear understanding of regimen.
• Discuss expected lag period (3–4 wk) before therapeutic ef-

fects can be anticipated.
• Review most common side effects: dry mouth, constipation, dizziness, urinary hesitancy, headache, nausea, sedation, or agitation, and encourage patient to report any side effects promptly.
• Caution patient against abrupt discontinuation without consulting prescriber. Abrupt discontinuation may cause withdrawal symptoms (cholinergic rebound, malaise, chills, coryza, muscle aches, agitation, insomnia) or rapid reemergence of depressive symptoms.
• Caution patient about ETOH or drug use.

METHYL-PHENIDATE HYDROCHLORIDE

Ritalin

PREGNANCY CATEGORY C

C-II controlled substance

Drug Classification: *Type:* CNS stimulant.

Mechanisms of Action
Mild cortical stimulant with CNS actions similar to those of the amphetamines. Efficacy in hyperkinetic syndrome, attention-deficit disorders in children appears paradoxical and is not completely understood.

Indications

Narcolepsy.

Attention deficit disorders, hyperkinetic syndrome, minimal brain dysfunction in children with a behavioral syndrome characterized by these symptoms: moderate to severe distractibility, short attention span, hyperactivity, emotional lability and impulsivity not secondary to environmental factors or psychiatric disorders.

Unlabeled uses: treatment of depression in the elderly; cancer and poststroke patients.

Contraindications/Cautions

Contraindications: • hypersensitivity to methylphenidate • marked anxiety, tension and agitation • glaucoma • motor tics, family history or diagnosis of Tourette's Syndrome • severe depression of endogenous or exogenous origin • normal fatigue states.

Use cautiously with: • seizure disorders • hypertension • drug dependence, alcoholism, emotional instability • lactation.

Dosage

Adult: Administer orally in divided doses bid–tid, preferably 30–45 min before meals. Dosage ranges from 10–60 mg/d. If insomnia is a problem, drug should be taken before 6 p.m.

Timed release tablets have a duration of 8 h and may be used when timing and dosage are titrated to the 8-h regimen.

Pediatric: Start with small oral doses, e.g., 5 mg PO, before breakfast and lunch with gradual increments of 5–10 mg weekly. Daily dosage >60 mg not recommended. Discontinue use after 1 mo if no improvement. Discontinue periodically to assess condition; usually discontinued after puberty.

Dosage Forms: Tablets: 5, 10, 20 mg; Sustained release tablets: 20 mg.

Pharmacokinetics

Absorption: rapidly from the GI tract. *Distribution:* crosses placenta and passes into breast milk. *Metabolism:* hepatic; $T_{1/2}$:1–3 h. *Peak levels:* 1–3 h. *Elimination:* urine.

Adverse Effects

CNS: Nervousness, insomnia, dizziness, headache, dyskinesia, chorea, drowsiness, Tourette's Syndrome, toxic psychosis, blurred vision, accommodation difficulties.

CV: Increased or decreased pulse and blood pressure; tachycardia, angina, cardiac arrhythmias, palpitations.

GI: Anorexia, nausea, abdominal pain; weight loss.

DERMATOLOGIC: Skin rash,

urticaria, fever, arthralgia, exfoliative dermatitis, erythema multiforme with necrotizing vasculitis and thrombocytopenic purpura, loss of scalp hair.

HEMATOLOGIC: Leukopenia, anemia.

OTHER: Tolerance, psychological dependence, abnormal behavior with abuse.

Clinically Important Drug–Drug Interactions

⧧ Decreased antihypertensive effect of guanethidine if taken together.
⧧ Possible increased serum levels of TCAs and phenytoin and increased risk of toxicity if combined.

Nursing Considerations

Assessment

• Assess for any of the conditions listed under "Contraindications/Cautions" above.
• Assess for history of alcohol or drug dependence or abuse, use of current prescription or OTC medications.
• Complete physical exam: vital signs, orientation, affect, ophthalmologic exam (tonometry), CBC with differential and platelet count, baseline ECG.
• Assure proper diagnosis before administering to children for behavioral syndromes: drug should not be used until other causes/concomitants of abnormal behavior (learning disability, EEG abnormalities, neurological deficits) are ruled out.
• Arrange to interrupt drug dosage periodically in children being treated for behavioral disorders to determine if symptoms recur at an intensity that warrants continued drug therapy.
• Monitor growth of children on long-term methylphenidate therapy.
• Arrange to monitor CBC, platelet counts periodically in patients on long-term therapy.

Drug-Specific Patient Education

• Review the target symptoms that the drug potentially treats: hyperactivity, attention deficit, falling asleep with no warning.
• Review the dosing schedule until patient and/or significant other demonstrates a clear understanding of regimen, including swallowing time-release tablets whole, taking drug before 6 p.m. to avoid nighttime sleep disturbances.
• Review the most common side effects: nervousness, restlessness, dizziness, insomnia, impaired thinking, headache, loss of appetite, dry mouth.
• Review the side effects patient should report promptly: nervousness, insomnia, palpitations, vomiting, skin rash, fever.
• Caution parents of pediatric

patients of need to stop drug to challenge effect and the need to monitor growth in these patients.
• Caution patient to avoid the use of alcohol and sleep inducing or OTC drugs.

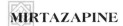

MIRTAZAPINE

REMERON
PREGNANCY CATEGORY B

Drug Classification: *Type:* antidepressant; *Class:* tetracyclic.

Mechanisms of Action
Appears to act similarly to the tricyclic antidepressants (TCAs). The TCAs act to inhibit the presynaptic reuptake of the neurotransmitters norepinephrine and serotonin; anticholinergic at CNS and peripheral receptors; sedating. The relation of these effects to clinical efficacy is unknown.

Indications
Relief of symptoms of depression (endogenous depression most responsive).

Contraindications/Cautions
Contraindications: • hypersensitivity to any tricyclic or tetracyclic drug • concomitant therapy with an MAO inhibitor • recent MI • myelography within previous 24 h or scheduled within 48 h • pregnancy (limb reduction abnormalities reported) • lactation.
Use cautiously with: • electroshock therapy • preexisting cardiovascular disorders (e.g., severe coronary heart disease, progressive heart failure, angina pectoris, paroxysmal tachycardia) • angle-closure glaucoma • increased intraocular pressure • urinary retention • ureteral or urethral spasm • seizure disorders • hyperthyroidism • impaired hepatic or renal function • psychiatric patients • elective surgery.

Dosage
Adult: Initial dose: 15 mg PO qd, as a single dose in the evening. Continue treatment for up to 6 mo for acute episodes. *Switching from an MAOI:* Allow at least 14 d between the discontinuation of the MAOI and the beginning of mirtazapine therapy. Allow 14 d after stopping mirtazapine before starting an MAOI.

Pediatric Adolescent: Not recommended in children <18 y of age.

Geriatric: Give lower doses to patients >60 y.

Dosage Forms: Tablets: 15, 30 mg.

Blood Levels: Utility has not been established.

Pharmacokinetics

Absorption: slowly from the GI tract. *Distribution:* plasma protein-bound; crosses placenta and enters breast milk. *Metabolism:* hepatic; $T_{1/2}$: 20–40 h. *Peak levels:* 5 h. *Steady state:* 5 d. *Excretion:* urine and feces.

Adverse Effects

CNS: Sedation and anticholinergic (atropine-like) effects; confusion (especially in elderly), disturbed concentration, hallucinations, disorientation, decreased memory, feelings of unreality, delusions, anxiety, nervousness, restlessness, agitation, panic, insomnia, nightmares, hypomania, mania, exacerbation of psychosis, drowsiness, weakness, fatigue, headache, numbness, agitation (less likely with this drug than other antidepressants).

GI: Dry mouth, constipation, paralytic ileus, nausea (less likely with this drug than other antidepressants), vomiting, anorexia, epigastric distress, diarrhea, flatulence, dysphagia, peculiar taste, increased salivation, stomatitis, glossitis, parotid swelling, abdominal cramps, black tongue, liver enzyme elevations.

GU: Urinary retention, delayed micturition, dilation of the urinary tract, gynecomastia, testicular swelling in men; breast enlargement, menstrual irregularity and galactorrhea in women; increased or decreased libido; impotence.

CV: Orthostatic hypotension, hypertension, syncope, tachycardia, palpitations, MI, arrhythmias, heart block, precipitation of CHF, stroke.

HEMATOLOGIC: Agranulocytosis, neutropenia.

ENDOCRINE: Elevated or depressed blood sugar; elevated prolactin levels; inappropriate ADH secretion.

HYPERSENSITIVITY: Skin rash, pruritus, vasculitis, petechiae, photosensitization, edema.

Nursing Considerations

Assessment

• Assess for any conditions listed under "Contraindications/Cautions" above.
• Assess for any ETOH and drug use and for concomitant prescribed and/or OTC medications.
• Assess for suicidal ideation.
• Complete physical exam: vital signs, skin color, lesions, orientation, affect, reflexes, usual sexual function, liver function tests, urinalysis, CBC, ECG.

Drug-Specific Patient Education

• Review the target symptoms that the drug potentially treats: depression.

• Review the dosing schedule until patient demonstrates a clear understanding of regimen.

• Review the expected lag period: 3–7 d for response, up to 2–3 wk for full effect.

• Review the most common side effects: headache, dizziness, drowsiness, weakness, blurred vision, nausea, vomiting, loss of appetite, dry mouth, nightmares, inability to concentrate, confusion, changes in sexual function, sensitivity to sunlight.

• Review the side effects patient should report promptly: fever, flu-like illness, any infection, dry mouth, difficulty in urination, excessive sedation.

• Caution patient to avoid the use of alcohol and sleep-inducing or OTC drugs.

MOLINDONE HYDROCHLORIDE

• •

Moban

PREGNANCY CATEGORY C

Drug Classification: *Type:* dopamine receptor antagonist; also called antipsychotic, neuroleptic, or major tranquilizer; *Class:* dihydroindole.

Mechanisms of Action

Postsynaptic antagonism of dopamine receptors, primarily D2 (antipsychotic efficacy is thought to be mediated by these actions). Blockade of muscarinic cholinergic, noradrenergic, and histaminergic receptors (some undesirable side effects are thought to be mediated by these actions).

Indications

Short- and long-term management of idiopathic psychoses including schizophrenia, schizophreniform disorder, schizoaffective disorder, delusional disorder, brief psychotic disorder, mania with psychosis, and major depressive disorder with psychotic features.

Secondary psychoses associated with a general medical condition or substance-related disorder.

Acute deliria and organic psychoses.

Severe agitation or violent behavior.

Severe behavioral problems in children marked by combativeness and/or explosive hyperexcitability and in the short-term treatment of hyperactive children who show excessive motor activity.

Movement disorder of Huntington's disease.

Motor and vocal tics of Tourette's Syndrome.

Brief use for episodes of severe

dyscontrol or apparent psychosis in some personality disorders.

Control of nausea, vomiting, and intractable hiccups.

Contraindications/Cautions

Contraindications: • allergy to molindone • comatose or severely depressed states • presence of large amounts of CNS depressants (alcohol, barbiturates, narcotics, etc.) • bone marrow depression • blood dyscrasias • circulatory collapse • subcortical brain damage • Parkinson's disease • liver damage • cerebral or coronary arteriosclerosis • CV disease • severe hypotension or hypertension • respiratory disorders • glaucoma • history of epilepsy or seizures • peptic ulcer or history of peptic ulcer • decreased renal function • urinary retention, ureteral or urethral spasm • prostate hypertrophy • breast cancer • thyrotoxicosis • myelography within 24 h or scheduled within 48 h • pregnancy • lactation • exposure to heat, organophosphorous insecticides, or atropine or related drugs • children with chickenpox • CNS infections • if signs and symptoms of tardive dyskinesia appear, drug discontinuation should be considered • history of neuroleptic malignant syndrome.

Dosage

Adult: Patients may respond to widely different dosages of antipsychotics. Therefore, there is no set dosage for any given antipsychotic drug. Usual range for acute use (oral): 50–250 mg/d. Usual range for maintenance use (oral): 10–200 mg/d. Can be administered once a day.

Pediatric Adolescent: Generally not used in children <12 y; >12 start at lowest adult dosage.

Geriatric: Start dosage at one-fourth to one-third that given in younger adults and increase more gradually.

Dosage Forms: Tablets: 5, 10, 25, 50, 100 mg; Liquid concentrate: 20 mg/ml.

Pharmacokinetics

Absorption: (oral) adequate but variable; food or antacids may decrease absorption; liquid preparations are absorbed more rapidly and reliably than tablets; onset of action 3–60 min; peak level: 2–4 h. *Distribution:* highly protein bound (85–90%) and lipophilic; readily crosses the blood–brain barrier, placenta, and enters breast milk; concentrations in the brain appear to be greater than those in blood; not removed efficiently by dialysis. *Metabolism:* hepatic. *Elimination:* urine. The elimination half-life of most antipsychotic drugs is 18–40 h; plasma levels may vary among individuals by 10- to 20-fold.

Adverse Effects

CNS: Drowsiness, insomnia, vertigo, headache, weakness, tremors, ataxia, slurring of speech, cerebral edema, seizures, exacerbation of psychotic symptoms, extrapyramidal syndromes (EPS), neuroleptic malignant syndrome, tardive dyskinesia, pseudo-parkinsonism, akathisia (see descriptions of symptoms under "Implementation" below).

GI: Dry mouth, salivation, nausea, vomiting, anorexia, constipation, paralytic ileus.

CV: Hypotension, orthostatic hypotension, hypertension, tachycardia, bradycardia, cardiac arrest, CHF, cardiomegaly, refractory arrhythmias, dysrhythmias, pulmonary edema.

RESPIRATORY: Bronchospasm, laryngospasm, dyspnea, suppression of cough reflex, and potential aspiration.

HEMATOLOGIC: Eosinophilia, leukopenia, leukocytosis, anemia, aplastic anemia, hemolytic anemia, thrombocytopenic or nonthrombocytopenic purpura, pancytopenia, elevated serum cholesterol.

GU: Urinary retention, polyuria, incontinence, priapism, ejaculation inhibition, male impotence, urine discolored pink to red-brown.

EENT: Nasal congestion, glaucoma, photophobia, blurred vision, miosis, mydriasis, deposits in the cornea and lens, pigmentary retinopathy.

HYPERSENSITIVITY: Jaundice, urticaria, angioneurotic edema, laryngeal edema, photosensitivity, eczema, asthma, anaphylactoid reactions, exfoliative dermatitis, contact dermatitis.

ENDOCRINE: Lactation, breast engorgement in females, galactorrhea, syndrome of inappropriate ADH secretion, amenorrhea, menstrual irregularities, gynecomastia, changes in libido, hyperglycemia, inhibition of ovulation, infertility, pseudopregnancy, reduced urinary levels of gonadotropins, estrogens, and progestins.

OTHER: Fever, heat stroke, pallor, flushed facies, sweating.

Clinically Important Drug–Drug Interactions

⧗ Additive anticholinergic effects and possibly decreased antipsychotic efficacy with anticholinergic drugs.
⧗ Additive CNS depression and hypotension with barbiturates, alcohol, meperidine.
⧗ Additive effects of both drugs with beta-blockers.
⧗ Increased risk of tachycardia,

hypotension with epinephrine, norepinephrine.

⇉ Increased risk of seizure with metrizamide.

⇉ Decreased hypotension effect with guanethidine.

⇉ Because of displacement and competition for protein binding sites, concomitant treatment with other highly protein-bound medications (e.g., warfarin, digoxin) could alter concentrations of both drugs.

⇉ Decreased effect of oral anticoagulants.

⇉ Possible increase in phenytoin levels.

Lab Test Interference

• False-positive pregnancy tests (less likely if serum test is used).

• Increase in protein-bound iodine, not attributable to an increase in thyroxine.

• Blood levels of antipsychotics have not correlated well with clinical response and serum levels are probably more misleading than useful.

Nursing Considerations

Assessment

• Assess for any of the conditions listed under "Contraindications/Cautions" above.

• Assess for alcohol and drug use/abuse and for concomitant use of prescription and/or OTC medications.

• Assess for risk of suicidality.

• Complete physical exam:

vital signs including orthostatic BP, ECG, CBC with differential, thyroid and liver function, BUN, creatinine.

Implementation

• Bioavailability differs between brand names of oral forms.

• Dilute liquid concentrate just before administration in 60 ml or more of fruit juice, milk, simple syrup, orange syrup, carbonated beverage, coffee, tea, water, or semisolid foods.

• Protect liquid concentrate from light.

• Be alert to potential for aspiration because of suppressed cough reflex.

• Monitor for dehydration, renal or liver abnormalities, depressed WBC, symptoms of infection. Promptly report to prescriber and institute remedial measures.

• Monitor for extrapyramidal side effects (involuntary dystonic muscular movements of the neck, jaw, tongue, or entire body; swallowing difficulties; oculogyric crisis); Parkinsonism (muscle stiffness; cogwheel rigidity; shuffling gait, stooped posture, drooling, coarse tremor, "rabbit syndrome," masklike facies, bradykinesia, akinesia); akathisia (subjective feeling of muscular discomfort that can cause agitation, restlessness, pacing, rocking, continually changing posture, and dysphoria).

• Monitor for symptoms of neuroleptic malignant syndrome: muscle rigidity; altered mental status; evidence of autonomic instability (e.g., irregular pulse or blood pressure, tachycardia, cardiac dysrhythmias); hyperpyrexia, sweating; increased WBC, blood creatinine phosphokinase, liver enzymes, myoglobin; mutism, obtundation, agitation.

• Monitor for symptoms of tardive dyskinesia (abnormal, involuntary, irregular, choreoathetoid movements of muscles of the head, limbs, and trunk; darting, twisting, and protruding movements of the tongue; chewing and lateral jaw movements; lip puckering; facial grimacing; finger movements and hand clenching; torticollis, retrocollis, trunk twisting, pelvic thrusting).

• Taper drug gradually after high-dose therapy due to possible gastritis, nausea, dizziness, headache, tachycardia, insomnia after abrupt withdrawal.

Drug-Specific Patient Education

• Review target symptoms that drug potentially treats: auditory, visual, olfactory, tactile hallucinations; delusions; paranoia; disorders of thought and speech; psychotic agitation; insomnia.

• Review dosing schedule until patient demonstrates a clear understanding of regimen. Caution patient against changing dosage or discontinuation without consulting prescriber.

• Caution patient against concurrent alcohol or drug use.

• Discuss expected lag period (6 wk or more) before full therapeutic effects appear.

• Review most common side effects (drowsiness, insomnia, dry mouth, constipation, dizziness from hypotension, urinary hesitancy or retention, photosensitivity, blurred vision, urticaria, EPS, Parkinsonism, akathisia), and encourage patient to report any side effects promptly.

• If possible, give the patient full information about the risk of tardive dyskinesia and possible irreversibility. (The decision whether to inform patients and/or their guardians must take into account the clinical circumstances and the competency of the patient to understand the information provided.)

• Educate patient about possibly life-threatening blood dyscrasias and instruct patient to report fever, chills, sore throat, unusual bleeding or bruising, or rash and to discontinue medication immediately (most likely between 4th and 10th weeks of treatment).

• Caution patient about risk of dehydration or heat stroke, increased risk of sunburn, and warn against over exercising in a hot climate.

NEFAZODONE HYDROCHLORIDE

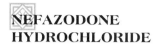

••••••••••••••••••••••••

Serzone

PREGNANCY CATEGORY C

Drug Classification: *Type:* serotonin transport inhibitor; antidepressant; phenylpiperazine analogue of trazodone.

Mechanisms of Action
Presynaptic serotonin reuptake inhibitor; postsynaptic serotonin antagonism; adrenergic receptor antagonism.

Indications
Treatment of major depression; anxiety symptoms and insomnia associated with depression; effective in improving sleep duration and quality; severe agitation in geriatric patients; premenstrual dysphoric disorder; pain management.

Contraindications/Cautions
Contraindications: • hypersensitivity to nefazodone • pregnancy • lactation • EST • recent MI • cardiac disease • risk of toxicity and serotonin syndrome with MAO inhibitor.
Use cautiously with: • hepatic or renal impairment • seizure history • may cause hypomania or mania.

Dosage
Adult: 100–600 mg qd. May be given qd or bid with major portion at hs. Consider trial a failure if patient shows no response on maximum recommended dose after 4–6 wk.

Pediatric Adolescent: Safety and efficacy not established for children <18 y.

Geriatric: Give smallest adult dose and increase slowly and cautiously.

Dosage Forms: Tablets: 100, 150, 200, 250 mg.

Pharmacokinetics
Absorption: readily absorbed from GI tract. *Distribution:* 99% protein-bound and widely distributed; crosses placenta, may enter breast milk. *Metabolism:* hepatic; peak plasma level 2–4 h; $T_{1/2}$: 11–24 h. *Elimination:* urine and feces.

Adverse Effects
CNS: Hypomania, confusion, dizziness, incoordination, somnolence, insomnia, nervousness, blurred vision, malaise, headache, lightheadedness.

CV: Hypertension, hypotension.

GI: Abdominal/gastric disorders, increased appetite, dry mouth, nausea, vomiting, diarrhea, constipation.

GU: Decreased libido and sexual function, increased urinary frequency/retention; vaginitis, breast pain.

SKIN: Pruritus, rash.

Clinically Important Drug–Drug Interactions

⚕ Increased risk of severe toxic effects with MAOIs, astemizole, terfenadine.

⚕ Increased levels of triazolam and alprazolam.

⚕ May increase digoxin levels.

Nursing Considerations

Assessment

• Assess for any of the conditions listed in "Contraindications/Cautions" above.

• Assess for concurrent prescription, OTC, or illegal drug or ETOH use/abuse; risk of suicide. Limit potentially suicidal patients' access to drug.

• Complete physical, vital signs, weight; CBC with differential; liver and thyroid function tests; BUN; creatinine; ECG if >40 y.

Drug-Specific Patient Education

• Review target symptoms that drug potentially treats: disruptions in sleep, appetite, concentration, energy, mood; anhedonia; interest; motivation; initiative; suicidal ideation, anxiety.

• Review dosing schedule until patient demonstrates a clear understanding of regimen.

• Discuss expected lag period (3–4 wk) before full therapeutic effects can be anticipated.

• Review most common side effects (sedation, dizziness, nausea, dry mouth, constipation, asthenia, lightheadedness, blurred vision, confusion, and abnormal vision) and encourage patient to report any side effects promptly.

• Educate patient about contraception during drug use.

• Caution patient about concurrent ETOH and drug use.

NORTRIPTYLINE HYDROCHLORIDE

Aventyl, Pamelor

PREGNANCY CATEGORY C

Drug Classification: *Type:* Antidepressant; *Class:* tricyclic (TCA); *Subclass:* secondary amine.

Mechanisms of Action

Presynaptic reuptake inhibition of neurotransmitters norepinephrine and serotonin (antidepressant efficacy is thought to be mediated by these actions). Postsynaptic blockade of histaminic, muscarinic, and noradrenergic alpha-one and alpha-two receptors (some of the undesirable side effects are thought to be mediated by these actions).

Indications

Relief of symptoms of depression (endogenous depression most responsive).

Unlabeled uses: relief of symptoms of anxiety and panic disorders; control of chronic pain.

Contraindications/Cautions

Contraindications: • hypersensitivity to any tricyclic drug • concomitant therapy with an MAO inhibitor • ECT with coadministration of TCAs • recent MI • myelography within previous 24 h or scheduled within 48 h.

Use cautiously with: • preexisting CV disorders, especially cardiac conduction system disease • seizure disorders • hyperthyroidism • angle-closure glaucoma • increased intraocular pressure • urinary retention • ureteral or urethral spasm • impaired hepatic or renal function • bipolar patients shifting to hypomanic or manic phase • elective surgery • pregnancy • lactation.

Dosage

Adult: Typical starting dose 25 mg qhs. Can be administered once a day, usually at hs, or in divided doses if patient has side effects due to high peak levels. Increase by 25 mg q 3–4 d as side effects allow. Usual maintenance dose 50–150 mg/d. Earliest onset of action in 2–5 d. Consider drug trial a failure if patient has been on maximal dose for 4–6 wk without response. Limit potentially suicidal patients' access to drug.

Pediatric Adolescent: Not recommended in children <12 y.

Geriatric: Initially 10 mg/d. Adjust dose according to tolerance and blood level.

Dosage Forms: Tablets: 10, 25, 50, 75 mg.

Blood Levels: Draw only to assess compliance; to confirm rapid or slow metabolizers; to document adequate drug trial. Therapeutic range: 50–150 ng/ml; greater than 150 ng/ml may reduce efficacy; levels should be drawn when any dose has reached steady state (5–7 d) and 10–14 h after last dose.

Pharmacokinetics

Absorption: from GI tract rapidly and completely. *Distribution:* highly lipophilic and largely protein bound; crosses blood–brain barrier and placenta and enters breast milk. *Metabolism:* hepatic; $T_{1/2}$: 48–72 h. *Elimination:* urine. *Steady state:* 5–7 d.

Adverse Effects

Adult Use

CNS: Sedation and anticholinergic effects—dry mouth, blurred vision, disturbance of accommodation for near vision, mydriasis, increased intraocular pressure; confusion, disturbed concentration, hallucinations, disorientation, decreased memory, feelings of unreality, delusions, anxiety, nervousness, restlessness, agitation, panic, insomnia, nightmares, hypomania, mania, exacerbation of psychosis, drowsiness, weakness, fatigue, headache, numbness, tingling, paresthesias of extremities, discoordination, motor hyperactivity, akathisia, ataxia, tremors, peripheral neuropathy, extrapyramidal symptoms, seizures, speech blockage, dysarthria, tinnitus, altered EEG.

GI: Dry mouth, constipation, paralytic ileus, nausea, vomiting, anorexia, epigastric distress, diarrhea, flatulence, dysphagia, peculiar taste, increased salivation, stomatitis, glossitis, parotid swelling, abdominal cramps, black tongue, hepatitis.

CV: Orthostatic hypotension, hypertension, syncope, tachycardia, palpitations, MI, arrhythmias, heart block, precipitation of CHF, stroke.

HEMATOLOGIC: Bone marrow depression, including agranulocytosis; eosinophilia, purpura, thrombocytopenia.

GU: Urinary retention, delayed micturition, dilation of the urinary tract, gynecomastia, testicular swelling in men; breast enlargement, menstrual irregularity, and galactorrhea in women; increased or decreased libido; impotence.

HYPERSENSITIVITY: Skin rash, pruritus, vasculitis, petechiae, photosensitization, edema (generalized, facial, tongue), drug fever.

ENDOCRINE: Elevated or depressed blood sugar, elevated prolactin levels, inappropriate ADH secretion.

WITHDRAWAL: Abrupt discontinuation of prolonged therapy: nausea, headache, vertigo, nightmares, malaise.

OTHER: Nasal congestion, excessive appetite, weight gain or loss; sweating (paradoxical effect in a drug with prominent anticholinergic effects), alopecia, lacrimation, hyperthermia, flushing, chills.

Clinically Important Drug–Drug Interactions

⊕ Increased sedation with alcohol, antihistamines, antipsychotics, barbiturates, chloral hydrate, and other sedatives.
⊕ Increased hypotension with alpha-methyldopa, beta-adrenergic blockers, clonidine, diuretics, low-potency antipsychotics.
⊕ Additive cardiotoxicity with quinidine and other class II antiarrhythmics, thioridazine,

mesoridazine, pimozide.

⇶ Additive anticholinergic toxicity with antihistamines, antiparkinsonians, low-potency antipsychotics, especially thioridazine, over-the-counter sleeping medications, gastrointestinal antispasmodics and antidiarrheals.

⇶ TCAs may increase the effects of warfarin and block the effects of guanethidine.

⇶ Increased sympathomimetic (especially alpha-adrenergic) effects of direct-acting sympathomimetic drugs (norepinephrine, epinephrine).

⇶ Decreased effects of indirect-acting sympathomimetic drugs (ephedrine).

⇶ Increased levels and possible delirium with disulfiram.

Note: MAOIs and TCAs have been used successfully in some patients who are resistant to therapy with single agents; however, hyperpyretic crises, severe convulsions, hypertensive episodes, and deaths can occur when MAOIs are given with TCAs.

Nursing Considerations

Assessment

• Assess for any of the conditions listed under "Contraindications/Cautions" above.

• Assess for ETOH or drug use/abuse and for concomitant prescribed and/or OTC medications.

• Assess for suicidal ideation.

• Complete physical exam: vital signs, EKG for patients 40 y or older, CBC with differential, thyroid function, liver function, BUN, creatinine, weight changes, I & O, vision; sexual interest, function, and activity.

Drug-Specific Patient Education

• Review target symptoms that drug potentially treats: disruptions in sleep, appetite, concentration, energy, mood; anhedonia; interest; motivation; initiative.

• Review dosing schedule until patient demonstrates a clear understanding of regimen.

• Discuss expected lag period (3–4 wk) before therapeutic effects can be anticipated.

• Review most common side effects: dry mouth, constipation, dizziness, urinary hesitancy, headache, nausea, sedation, or agitation, and encourage patient to report any side effects promptly.

• Caution patient against abrupt discontinuation without consulting prescriber. Abrupt discontinuation may cause withdrawal symptoms (cholinergic rebound, malaise, chills, coryza, muscle aches, agitation, insomnia) or rapid reemergence of depressive symptoms.

• Caution patient about ETOH or drug use.

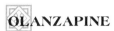 OLANZAPINE

· ·

Zyprexa

PREGNANCY CATEGORY C

Drug Classification: *Type:* antipsychotic; *Class:* dopaminergic blocker; *Subclass:* thienbenzodiazepine.

Mechanisms of Action

Blocks dopamine receptors in the brain, depresses the reticular activating system; blocks serotonin receptor sites. Anticholinergic, antihistaminic (H1), and alpha-adrenergic blocker, which may contribute to some of its therapeutic (and adverse) actions. Olanzapine produces fewer extrapyramidal effects than most antipsychotics; mechanism of action not fully understood.

Indications

Management of the manifestations of schizophrenia and psychotic disorders.

Contraindications/Cautions

Contraindications: • allergy to olanzapine • myeloproliferative disorders • severe CNS depression • comatose states • history of seizure disorders • lactation.
  Use cautiously with:
• cardiovascular or cerebrovascular disease • dehydration • seizure disorders • Alzheimer's disease • prostate enlargement • narrow-angle glaucoma • history of paralytic ileus or breast cancer • the elderly or debilitated • pregnancy.

Dosage

Adult: Initially 5–10 mg PO qd; increase to 10 mg PO qd within several days; may be increased by 5 mg/d at 1 wk intervals to achieve desired effect. Do not exceed 20 mg/d.

Pediatric Adolescent: Safety and efficacy in children <18 y not established.

Dosage Forms: Tablets: 5, 7.5, 10 mg.

Pharmacokinetics

Absorption: rapidly from the GI tract. *Distribution:* highly plasma protein-bound; widely distributed; crosses placenta and passes into breast milk. *Metabolism:* hepatic; $T_{1/2}$: 8–12 h. *Peak levels:* 6. *Steady state:* 1–2 wk. *Elimination:* urine and feces.

Adverse Effects

  CNS: Somnolence, dizziness, nervousness, headache, akathisia, personality disorders, tardive dyskinesia, Neuroleptic Malignant Syndrome.

  CV: Postural hypotension, peripheral edema, tachycardia.

  GI: Constipation, abdominal pain.

  RESPIRATORY: Cough, pharyngitis.

OTHER: Fever, weight gain, joint pain.

Clinically Important Drug–Drug Interactions

⇇ Increased risk of orthostatic hypotension with antihypertensives, alcohol, benzodiazepines.
⇇ Increased risk of seizures when combined with anticholinergics, CNS drugs.
⇇ May decrease the effectiveness of levodopa, dopamine agonists.
⇇ Decreased effectiveness of olanzapine if combined with rifampin, omeprazole, carbamazepine, smoking.
⇇ Increased risk of toxicity if combined with fluvoxamine.

Nursing Considerations

Assessment
• Assess for any conditions listed under "Contraindications/Cautions" above.
• Assess for history or alcohol or drug abuse or dependence, use of current prescribed or OTC medications.
• Complete physical exam: vital signs, orthostatic BP, reflexes, orientation, intraocular pressure, CBC, urinalysis, liver and kidney function tests.
• Assess any elevations of temperature and differentiate between infection and neuroleptic malignant syndrome.

• Assess elderly patients for dehydration, and institute remedial measures promptly—sedation and decreased sensation of thirst related to CNS effects of drug can lead to dehydration.

Drug-Specific Patient Education
• Review the target symptoms that the drug potentially treats: manifestations of schizophrenia and psychotic disorders.
• Review the dosing schedule until patient demonstrates a clear understanding of regimen.
• Review the most common side effects: drowsiness, dizziness, sedation, seizures; dizziness, faintness on arising; increased salivation; fast heart rate.
• Review the side effects patient should report promptly: lethargy, weakness, fever, sore throat, malaise, mouth ulcers, and "flu-like" symptoms.
• Caution patient to avoid pregnancy, use of barrier contraceptives is advised.
• Caution patient to avoid the use of alcohol and sleep-inducing or OTC drugs.

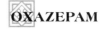OXAZEPAM

Apo-Oxazepam (CAN), Novoxapam (CAN), Ox-Pam (CAN), Serax, Zapex (CAN)

PREGNANCY CATEGORY D

C-IV controlled substance

Drug Classification: *Type:* anxiolytic; *Class:* 3-hydroxy-benzodiazepine.

Mechanisms of Action

Benzodiazepines bind to specific receptor sites associated with the major inhibitory neurotransmitter in the brain, gamma-aminobutyric acid (GABA), thereby increasing the affinity of the receptor sites. While the exact mechanisms of action are not completely understood, inhibitory actions on neurons within the limbic system, and on serotonergic (5-HT) and noradrenergic neurons within the brainstem, are responsible for the anxiolytic properties.

Indications

Relief of symptoms of anxiety. Symptomatic relief of acute alcohol withdrawal.

Contraindications/Cautions

Contraindications:
• hypersensitivity to benzodiazepines • psychoses, acute narrow-angle glaucoma, shock, coma, acute alcoholic intoxication • pregnancy (cleft lip or palate, inguinal hernia, cardiac defects, microcephaly, pyloric stenosis when used in first trimester; neonatal withdrawal syndrome reported in babies) • lactation.
Use cautiously with: • patients with history of alcohol or drug dependence or addiction
• elderly or debilitated patients
• patients with impaired liver or kidney function.

Dosage

Adult: 30–120 mg/d; may be given bid–qid.

Pediatric Adolescent: <12 y dosage not established.

Geriatric: Initial dose 10 mg/d; adjust dose according to tolerance and remission of symptoms.

Dosage Forms: Tablets: 15 mg; Capsules: 10, 15, 30 mg.

Pharmacokinetics

Absorption: from GI tract at slow rate with rapid onset of action. *Distribution:* highly lipid soluble, crosses placenta, passes into breast milk. *Metabolism:* hepatic; $T_{1/2}$: 10–30 h. *Peak plasma level:* 2–4 h. *Steady state:* up to 1 wk. *Elimination:* urine.

Adverse Effects

CNS: Transient, mild drowsiness initially; sedation, fatigue, ataxia; confusion, depression, lethargy, stupor, apathy, lightheadedness, disorientation, dysarthria, headache, slurred speech, tremor, vertigo, diplopia, nystagmus, paradoxical excitatory reactions, anxiety, hallucinations, euphoria, difficulty in concentration, vivid dreams, psychomotor retardation increased muscle spasticity, insomnia, rage, sleep disturbances, minor changes in EEG patterns.

GI: Constipation, changes in salivation, nausea, anorexia, vomiting, difficulty in swallowing, elevations of blood enzymes—LDH, alkaline phosphatase, SGOT, SGPT; hepatic dysfunction, jaundice.

CV: Bradycardia, tachycardia, hypertension and hypotension, palpitations, edema.

HEMATOLOGIC: Neutropenia, blood dyscrasias.

GU: Incontinence, urinary retention, changes in libido.

DERMATOLOGIC: Skin rashes.

TOLERANCE/DEPENDENCE: Some patients report a tolerance to the anxiolytic effects of benzodiazepines and require increased doses to maintain clinical remission. There is also a cross-tolerance among most of the benzodiazepines. Abrupt discontinuation, particularly of those with short half-lives, is associated with severe withdrawal symptoms seen only in patients who have taken high doses for long periods. Appearance of the syndrome may be delayed for 1–2 wk with benzodiazepines with very long half-lives. Commonly observed withdrawal symptoms in benzodiazepine withdrawal syndrome: anxiety, irritability, insomnia, fatigue, headache, muscle twitching or aching, tremor, shakiness, sweating, dizziness, concentration difficulties, nausea, anorexia, observable depression, depersonalization, derealization, increased sensory perception, abnormal perception or sensation of movement.

Clinically Important Drug–Drug Interactions

⌇ Decreased absorption with antacids.

⌇ Increased CNS depression with antihistamines, barbiturates and similarly acting drugs, cyclic antidepressants, alcohol, omeprazole.

⌇ Increased benzodiazepine level with cimetidine, disulfiram, erythromycin, estrogens, fluoxetine, isoniazid.

⌇ Decreased benzodiazepine levels with carbamazepine and, possibly, other anticonvulsants, theophyllines, ranitidine.

Nursing Considerations

Assessment

• Assess for any of the conditions listed under "Contraindications/Cautions" above.

• Assess for current use or history of alcohol or drug dependence or abuse, use of concurrent prescribed or OTC medications.

• Patient should have had routine complete physical within last year.

• Monitor vital signs during acute alcohol withdrawal; liver and kidney function; CBC with differential during long-term therapy.

• If discontinuing, taper dosage gradually (25% per week) and monitor for withdrawal symptoms.

Drug-Specific Patient Education

• Review symptoms specific to individual patient which drug potentially treats (anxiety, alcohol withdrawal, panic, phobias, insomnia).

• Review dosing schedule until patient demonstrates a clear understanding of regimen.

• Discuss expected onset of action.

• Review most common side effects (drowsiness, fatigue, ataxia) and encourage patient to report any side effects promptly.

• Caution patient about possible tolerance and/or psychological and physical dependence.

• Warn against abrupt discontinuation.

• Review possible withdrawal symptoms (see above under "Tolerance/Dependence").

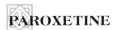

PAROXETINE

Paxil

PREGNANCY CATEGORY B

Drug Classification: *Type:* specific serotonin reuptake inhibitor (SSRI); antidepressant; *Class:* phenylpiperidine derivative.

Mechanisms of Action

Antidepressant activity associated with presynaptic reuptake of serotonin; no significant effects on norepinephrine, dopamine, or on adrenergic, histaminergic, and serotonergic receptors; unlike other SSRIs, paroxetine does have some anticholinergic effects.

Indications

Treatment of depression, panic disorder, dysthymia, eating disorders, obsessive-compulsive disorder (OCD).

Contraindications/Cautions

Contraindications: • hypersensitivity to paroxetine • MAO inhibitor use • pregnancy • lactation.

Use cautiously with: • impaired hepatic or renal function.

Dosage

Adult: 10–60 mg/d. May be given qd, usually in a.m. Earliest onset of action within 2–5 d. Consider drug trial a failure if patient has been on maximum recommended dose for 4–6 wk without response.

Pediatric Adolescent: Start at one-half the adult dose and increase slowly and cautiously.

Geriatric: Start at one-half the adult dose and increase slowly and cautiously.

Dosage Forms: Tablets: 20, 30 mg.

Pharmacokinetics

Absorption: from the GI tract; reaches peak plasma levels in 5 h. *Distribution:* 95% protein bound; lipophilic properties with wide tissue distribution; crosses placenta, enters breast milk. *Metabolism:* hepatic; $T_{1/2}$: 24 h. *Steady state:* 5–14 d. *Elimination:* urine.

Adverse Effects

CNS: Headaches, nervousness, insomnia, drowsiness, anxiety, tremor, dizziness, fatigue, sedation, sensation disturbance, decreased libido, light-headedness, decreased concentration.

GI: Nausea, diarrhea, dry mouth, anorexia, dyspepsia, constipation, abdominal pain, vomiting, taste change, flatulence, gastroenteritis.

SKIN: Excessive sweating, rash, pruritus.

BODY AS A WHOLE: Asthenia, viral infection, chest and limb pain, fever.

RESPIRATORY: Yawns, flu-like syndrome, pharyngitis.

CV: Hot flashes, palpitations, postural hypotension, hypertension.

MUSCULOSKELETAL: Back, joint, and muscle pain.

GU: Painful menstruation, sexual dysfunction, urinary frequency.

Clinically Important Drug–Drug Interactions

⊣ Toxic reactions or serotonin syndrome may occur with MAOIs or L-tryptophan.
⊣ When paroxetine is used with warfarin, bleeding time is increased; prothrombin time should be closely monitored.
⊣ Phenytoin may decrease levels of paroxetine.

Nursing Considerations

Assessment

• Assess for any of the conditions listed in "Contraindications/Cautions" above.
• Assess for concurrent prescription, OTC, or illegal drug or ETOH use/abuse, risk of suicide, and limit drug access to potentially suicidal patients.
• Complete physical, vital

signs, weight; CBC with differential; liver and thyroid function tests; BUN; creatinine; ECG if >40 y.

Drug-Specific Patient Education

• Review target symptoms that drug potentially treats: disruptions in sleep, appetite, concentration, energy, mood; anhedonia; interest; motivation; initiative; suicidal ideation, panic, obsessions, compulsions.
• Review dosing schedule until patient demonstrates a clear understanding of regimen.
• Discuss expected lag period (3–4 wk) before full therapeutic effects can be anticipated.
• Review most common side effects (agitation, anxiety, dizziness, insomnia, nausea, sweating, anorexia, diarrhea, tremor) and encourage patient to report any side effects promptly.
• Educate patient about contraception during drug use.
• Caution patient about concurrent ETOH and drug use.

PEMOLINE

• •

Cylert

PREGNANCY CATEGORY B

C-IV controlled substance

Drug Classification: *Type:* CNS stimulant.

Mechanisms of Action

CNS actions are similar to those of the amphetamines and methylphenidate, but has minimal sympathomimetic effects. May act through dopaminergic mechanisms. Efficacy in hyperkinetic syndrome, attention-deficit disorders in children appears paradoxical and is not understood.

Indications

Attention deficit disorders, hyperkinetic syndrome, minimal brain dysfunction in children with a behavioral syndrome characterized by these symptoms: moderate to severe distractibility, short attention span, hyperactivity, emotional lability and impulsivity, not secondary to environmental factors or psychiatric disorders (as part of a total treatment program).
Unlabeled use: Narcolepsy and excessive daytime sleepiness.

Contraindications/Cautions

Contraindications: • hypersensitivity to pemoline. impaired hepatic function.
  Use cautiously with: • impaired renal function • psychosis in children • epilepsy • drug dependence • alcoholism • emotional instability • lactation.

Dosage

Adult and Pediatric >6 y: Administer as a single oral dose each morning. Recommended starting dose is 37.5 mg/d. Gradually increase at 1 wk intervals using increments of 18.75 mg until desired response is obtained. Mean effective dose range is 56.25–75 mg/d. Do not exceed 112.5 mg/d.

Narcolepsy: 50–200 mg PO in two divided doses daily.

Pediatric: Not recommended in children <6 y.

Dosage Forms: Tablets: 18.75, 37.5, 75 mg; Chewable tablets: 37.5 mg.

Pharmacokinetics

Absorption: rapidly from the GI tract. *Distribution:* widely distributed, including the brain; crosses placenta and passes into breast milk. *Metabolism:* hepatic; $T_{1/2}$: 12 h. *Peak levels:* 2–4 h. *Steady state:* 2–3 d. *Elimination:* urine.

Adverse Effects

CNS: Insomnia, anorexia with weight loss (most common), dyskinetic movements of tongue, lips, face and extremities; Tourette's Syndrome; nystagmus; oculogyric crisis; convulsive seizures; increased irritability; mild depression; dizziness; headache; drowsiness; hallucinations.

GI: Stomachache, nausea, hepatitis; elevations of SGOT, SGPT, LDH; jaundice.

DERMATOLOGIC: Skin rashes.

OTHER: Aplastic anemia; tolerance, psychological or physical dependence.

Nursing Considerations

Assessment

• Assess for any conditions listed under "Contraindications/Cautions" above.

• Assess for history of alcohol or drug dependence/abuse, use of current prescribed or OTC medications.

• Complete physical exam: vital signs, orientation, affect, reflexes, CBC with differential, liver and kidney function tests.

• Assure proper diagnosis before administering to children for behavioral syndromes: drug should not be used until other causes/concomitants of abnormal behavior (learning disability, EEG abnormalities, neurological deficits) are ruled out.

• Arrange to interrupt drug dosage periodically in children being treated for behavioral disorders to determine if symptoms recur at an intensity that warrants continued drug therapy.

• Monitor growth of children.

• Arrange to monitor liver function tests periodically in patients on long-term therapy.

Drug-Specific Patient Education
• Review the target symptoms that the drug potentially treats: hyperactivity, attention deficit, sleepiness, falling asleep without warning.
• Review the dosing schedule until patient and/or significant other demonstrates a clear understanding of regimen.
• Review the most common side effects: insomnia, nervousness, restlessness, dizziness, impaired thinking; diarrhea; headache, loss of appetite, weight loss.
• Review the side effects patient should report promptly: insomnia, abnormal body movements, skin rash, severe diarrhea, pale color stools, yellowing of the skin or eyes.
• Caution parents of pediatric patients of need to stop drug to challenge effect and the need to monitor growth in these patients.
• Caution patient to avoid the use of alcohol and sleep inducing or OTC drugs.

PERPHENAZINE

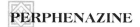

Apo-Perphenazine (CAN), Phenazine (CAN), Trilafon

PREGNANCY CATEGORY C

Drug Classification: *Type:* dopamine receptor antagonist; also called antipsychotic, neuroleptic, or major tranquilizer; *Class:* phenothiazine; *Subclass:* piperazine.

Mechanisms of Action
Postsynaptic antagonism of dopamine receptors, primarily D2 (antipsychotic efficacy is thought to be mediated by these actions). Blockade of muscarinic cholinergic, noradrenergic, and histaminergic receptors (some undesirable side effects are thought to be mediated by these actions).

Indications
Short- and long-term management of idiopathic psychoses including schizophrenia, schizophreniform disorder, schizoaffective disorder, delusional disorder, brief psychotic disorder, mania with psychosis, and major depressive disorder with psychotic features.

Secondary psychoses associated with a general medical condition or substance-related disorder.

Acute deliria and organic psychoses.

Severe agitation or violent behavior.

Severe behavioral problems in children marked by combativeness and/or explosive hyperexcitability and in the short-term treatment of hyperactive children who show excessive motor activity.

Movement disorder of Huntington's disease.

Motor and vocal tics of Tourette's Syndrome.

Brief use for episodes of severe dyscontrol or apparent psychosis in some personality disorders.

Control of nausea, vomiting, and intractable hiccups.

Contraindications/Cautions

Contraindications: • allergy to perphenazine; comatose or severely depressed states • presence of large amounts of CNS depressants (alcohol, barbiturates, narcotics, etc.) • bone marrow depression • blood dyscrasias • circulatory collapse • subcortical brain damage • Parkinson's disease • liver damage • cerebral or coronary arteriosclerosis • CV disease • severe hypotension or hypertension • respiratory disorders • glaucoma • history of epilepsy or seizures • peptic ulcer or history of peptic ulcer • decreased renal function • urinary retention, ureteral or urethral spasm • prostate hypertrophy • breast cancer • thyrotoxicosis • myelography within 24 h or scheduled within 48 h • pregnancy • lactation • exposure to heat, organophosphorous insecticides, or atropine or related

drugs • children with chickenpox • CNS infections • if signs and symptoms of tardive dyskinesia appear, drug discontinuation should be considered • history of neuroleptic malignant syndrome.

Dosage

Adult: Patients may respond to widely different dosages of antipsychotics. Therefore, there is no set dosage for any given antipsychotic drug. Usual range for acute use (oral): 8–32 mg/d. Usual range for maintenance use (oral): 8–24 mg/d. Can be administered once a day. IM: oral forms should be used whenever possible, but IM forms may be necessary for patients who exhibit violent behavior or for those who have high first-pass or presystemic metabolism of oral forms. Starting dose 5 mg IM; may repeat in 1 h; increase dosage gradually up to 30 mg/d. Switch to oral dosage as soon as patient is able or willing.

Pediatric Adolescent: Generally not used in children <12 y. >12 y may receive lowest adult dosage.

Geriatric: Start dosage at one-fourth to one-third that given in younger adults and increase more gradually.

Dosage Forms: Tablets: 2, 4, 8, 16 mg; Liquid concentrate: 16

mg/5 ml; 100 mg/ml; Injection: 5 mg/ml.

Pharmacokinetics

Absorption: (oral) adequate but variable; food or antacids may decrease absorption; liquid preparations are absorbed more rapidly and reliably than tablets; onset of action 3–60 min; peak level: 2–4 h; IM rapidly and reliably absorbed; onset of action 15–20 min; peak: 30–60 min. *Distribution:* highly protein bound (85–90%) and lipophilic; readily crosses the blood–brain barrier, placenta, and enters breast milk; concentrations in the brain appear to be greater than those in blood; not removed efficiently by dialysis. *Metabolism:* hepatic. *Elimination:* urine. The elimination half-life of most antipsychotic drugs is 18–40 h; plasma levels may vary among individuals by 10- to 20-fold.

Adverse Effects

CNS: Drowsiness, insomnia, vertigo, headache, weakness, tremors, ataxia, slurring of speech, cerebral edema, seizures, exacerbation of psychotic symptoms, extrapyramidal syndromes (EPS), neuroleptic malignant syndrome, tardive dyskinesia, pseudoparkinsonism, akathisia (see descriptions of symptoms under "Implementation" below).

GI: Dry mouth, salivation, nausea, vomiting, anorexia, constipation, paralytic ileus.

CV: Hypotension, orthostatic hypotension, hypertension, tachycardia, bradycardia, cardiac arrest, CHF, cardiomegaly, refractory arrhythmias, dysrhythmias, pulmonary edema.

RESPIRATORY: Bronchospasm, laryngospasm, dyspnea, suppression of cough reflex, and potential aspiration.

HEMATOLOGIC: Eosinophilia, leukopenia, leukocytosis, anemia, aplastic anemia, hemolytic anemia, thrombocytopenic or nonthrombocytopenic purpura, pancytopenia, elevated serum cholesterol.

GU: Urinary retention, polyuria, incontinence, priapism, ejaculation inhibition, male impotence, urine discolored pink to red-brown.

EENT: Nasal congestion, glaucoma, photophobia, blurred vision, miosis, mydriasis, deposits in the cornea and lens, pigmentary retinopathy.

HYPERSENSITIVITY: Jaundice, urticaria, angioneurotic edema, laryngeal edema, photosensitivity, eczema, asthma, anaphylactoid reactions, exfoliative dermatitis, contact dermatitis.

ENDOCRINE: Lactation, breast engorgement in females, galactorrhea, syndrome of inappropriate ADH secretion, amenorrhea, menstrual irregularities, gynecomastia, changes in libido, hyperglycemia, inhibition of ovulation, infertility, pseudopregnancy, reduced urinary levels of gonadotropins, estrogens, and progestins.

OTHER: Fever, heat stroke, pallor, flushed facies, sweating.

Clinically Important Drug–Drug Interactions

� Additive anticholinergic effects and possibly decreased antipsychotic efficacy with anticholinergic drugs.

� Additive CNS depression and hypotension with barbiturates, alcohol, meperidine.

� Additive effects of both drugs with beta-blockers.

� Increased risk of tachycardia, hypotension with epinephrine, norepinephrine.

� Increased risk of seizure with metrizamide.

� Decreased hypotensive effect with guanethidine.

� Because of displacement and competition for protein-binding sites, concomitant treatment with other highly protein-bound medications (e.g., warfarin, digoxin) could alter concentrations of both drugs.

� Decreased effect of oral anticoagulants.

� Possible increase in phenytoin levels.

Lab Test Interference

• False-positive pregnancy tests (less likely if serum test is used).

• Increase in protein-bound iodine not attributable to an increase in thyroxine.

• Blood levels of antipsychotics have not correlated well with clinical response and serum levels are probably more misleading than useful.

Nursing Considerations

Assessment

• Assess for any of the conditions listed under "Contraindications/Cautions" above.

• Assess for alcohol and drug use/abuse and for concomitant use of prescription and/or OTC medications.

• Assess for risk of suicidality.

• Complete physical exam: vital signs including orthostatic BP, ECG, CBC with differential, thyroid and liver function, BUN, creatinine.

Implementation

• Bioavailability differs between brand names of oral forms.

• Dilute liquid concentrate just before administration in 60 ml or more of fruit juice, milk, simple syrup, orange syrup, carbonated beverage, coffee, tea, water, or semisolid foods.

• Protect liquid concentrate from light.

• Give IM injection slowly into

upper outer-quadrant of buttock.
• Be alert to potential for aspiration because of suppressed cough reflex.
• Monitor for dehydration, renal or liver abnormalities, depressed WBC, symptoms of infection. Promptly report to prescriber and institute remedial measures.
• Monitor for extrapyramidal side effects (involuntary dystonic muscular movements of the neck, jaw, tongue, or entire body; swallowing difficulties; oculogyric crisis); Parkinsonism (muscle stiffness; cogwheel rigidity; shuffling gait, stooped posture, drooling, coarse tremor, "rabbit syndrome," masklike facies, bradykinesia, akinesia); akathisia (subjective feeling of muscular discomfort that can cause agitation, restlessness, pacing, rocking, continually changing posture, and dysphoria).
• Monitor for symptoms of Neuroleptic Malignant Syndrome: muscle rigidity; altered mental status; evidence of autonomic instability (e.g., irregular pulse or blood pressure, tachycardia, cardiac dysrhythmias); hyperpyrexia, sweating; increased WBC, blood creatinine phosphokinase, liver enzymes, myoglobin; mutism, obtundation, agitation.
• Monitor for symptoms of tardive dyskinesia (abnormal, involuntary, irregular, choreoathetoid movements of muscles of the head, limbs, and trunk; darting, twisting, and protruding movements of the tongue; chewing and lateral jaw movements; lip puckering; facial grimacing; finger movements and hand clenching; torticollis, retrocollis, trunk twisting, pelvic thrusting).
• Taper drug gradually after high-dose therapy due to possible gastritis, nausea, dizziness, headache, tachycardia, insomnia after abrupt withdrawal.

Drug-Specific Patient Education
• Review target symptoms that drug potentially treats: auditory, visual, olfactory, tactile hallucinations; delusions; paranoia; disorders of thought and speech; psychotic agitation; insomnia.
• Review dosing schedule until patient demonstrates a clear understanding of regimen. Caution patient against changing dosage or discontinuation without consulting prescriber.
• Caution patient against concurrent alcohol or drug use.
• Discuss expected lag period (6 wk or more) before full therapeutic effects appear.
• Review most common side effects (drowsiness, insomnia, dry mouth, constipation, dizziness from hypotension, urinary hesitancy or retention, photo-

sensitivity, blurred vision, urticaria, EPS, Parkinsonism, akathisia), and encourage patient to report any side effects promptly.
• If possible, give the patient full information about the risk of tardive dyskinesia and possible irreversibility. (The decision whether to inform patients and/or their guardians must take into account the clinical circumstances and the competency of the patient to understand the information provided.)
• Educate patient about possibly life-threatening blood dyscrasias and instruct patient to report fever, chills, sore throat, unusual bleeding or bruising, or rash and to discontinue medication immediately (most likely between 4th and 10th weeks of treatment).
• Caution patient about risk of dehydration or heat stroke, increased risk of sunburn, and warn against over exercising in a hot climate.

PHENELZINE SULFATE

· ·

Nardil

PREGNANCY CATEGORY C

Drug Classification: *Type:* antidepressant; monoamine oxidase inhibitor (MAOI); *Class:* hydrazine derivative.

Mechanisms of Action
Inhibition of the enzyme monoamine oxidase that breaks down the neurotransmitters serotonin and norepinephrine, thereby increasing their accumulation and availability (this action is believed to be responsible for antidepressant effect).

Indications
Treatment of major depression and atypical depression, panic, agoraphobia, posttraumatic stress disorder, eating disorders, social phobia, pain syndromes.

Contraindications/Cautions
Contraindications: • hypersensitivity to a MAOI
• pheochromocytoma • CHF
• history of liver disease or abnormal liver function • severe renal impairment • confirmed or suspected cerebrovascular defect • CV disease • hypertension • history of headache
• myelography within previous 24 h or scheduled within 48 h.
Use cautiously with:
• seizure disorders • hyperthyroidism • impaired hepatic or renal function • may cause hypomania or mania • patients scheduled for elective surgery
• pregnancy • lactation.

Dosage

Adult: 15–90 mg/d. Given bid or tid. Consider trial a failure if patient does not respond to maximum dose after 3–6 wk.

Pediatric Adolescent: Not recommended for children <16 y.

Geriatric: Start at lowest adult dosage and increase slowly and cautiously.

Dosage Forms: Tablets: 15 mg.

Pharmacokinetics

Absorption: readily absorbed from GI tract. *Distribution:* crosses placenta, enters breast milk. *Metabolism:* hepatic acetylation (a high percentage of Asians and about 50% of whites and blacks are slow acetylators and may have more adverse effects); $T_{1/2}$: unknown; maximal inhibition of MAO occurs after 5–10 d. *Elimination:* urine.

MAO Blood Levels

Although plasma levels of MAOIs are not well studied, the degree of enzyme inhibition produced has been investigated. Inhibition of greater than 85% of baseline platelet MAO type B activity appears to correlate with therapeutic efficacy. (Dosages >45 mg/d are usually necessary to achieve this level of inhibition.)

Adverse Effects

CNS: Dizziness, vertigo, headache, overactivity, tremors, muscle twitching, jitteriness, insomnia, anxiety, agitation, hyperflexia, hypomania, mania, confusion, memory impairment, weakness, fatigue, drowsiness, restlessness, overstimulation, blurred vision, sweating, akathisia, ataxia, coma, euphoria, neuritis.

GI: Constipation, diarrhea, nausea, abdominal pain, dry mouth, anorexia, weight changes, edema.

GU: Dysuria, incontinence, urinary retention, sexual disturbances.

SKIN: Minor skin reactions, spider telangiectases, photosensitivity.

OTHER: Hematologic changes, black tongue, hypernatremia.

CV: Hypertensive crisis usually attributable to ingestion of contraindicated food or drink containing tyramine (see "Clinically Important Drug–Food Interactions" below); symptoms include: hypertension, occipital headache, palpitations, neck stiffness or soreness; nausea; vomiting; sweating; dilated pupils; photophobia; tachycardia or bradycardia; chest pain, orthostatic hypotension, sometimes associated with falling; disturbed cardiac rate and rhythm.

Clinically Important Drug–Drug Interactions

⊣ Increased sympathomimetic effects (and possible hypertensive crisis) with sympathomimetic drugs (norepinephrine, epinephrine, dopamine, dobutamine, levodopa, ephedrine), amphetamines, other anorexians, local anesthetic solutions containing sympathomimetics.

⊣ Any serotonergic or noradrenergic antidepressant should be discontinued 7–10 d (3 wk for fluoxetine) before starting a MAOI or not started until 2 wk after discontinuing a MAOI.

⊣ Risk of hypertensive crisis, coma, severe convulsions with TCAs.

⊣ Additive hypoglycemic effect with insulin, oral sulfonylureas.

⊣ Increased risk of adverse interaction with meperidine.

Note: MAOIs and TCAs have been used successfully in some patients who are resistant to therapy with single agents.

Clinically Important Drug–Food Interactions

The amino acid tyramine are normally broken down by MAO in the GI tract. In the presence of MAOIs, tyramine, which is a vasopressor, may be absorbed in high concentrations and may release accumulated norepinephrine from nerve terminals. A hypertensive crisis may occur when the following foods, which contain tyramine, are ingested by a patient on a MAOI and, therefore, are contraindicated: Meat: beef liver, chicken liver, fermented sausages (pepperoni, salami, bologna, and others), other cured or unrefrigerated meats; Fish: caviar, cured, unrefrigerated fish, dried or pickled herring, dried fish, shrimp paste; Vegetables: overripe avocados, fava beans, sauerkraut; Fruits: overripe fruits, canned figs; yeast extracts (e.g., Marmite, Bovril); Chianti wine, beers containing yeast. Foods and beverages that should be used only in moderation: chocolate, caffeine, beer, wine. Medications to be avoided: all over-the-counter pain medications except plain aspirin, acetaminophen (Tylenol), and ibuprofen; all cold or allergy medications except plain chlorpheniramine (Chlor-Trimeton) or brompheniramine (Dimetane); all nasal decongestants and inhalers; all cough medications except plain guaifenesin elixir (plain Robitussin); all stimulants and diet pills.

Nursing Considerations

Assessment

• Assess for any of the conditions listed in "Contraindications/Cautions" above.

• Assess for concurrent prescription, OTC, or illegal drug or ETOH use/abuse; risk of suicide. Limit potentially suicidal patients' access to drug.

• Complete physical, vital signs, weight; CBC with differential; liver and thyroid function tests; BUN; creatinine; ECG if >40 y.

Implementation

• Monitor BP and orthostatic BP carefully and watch for symptoms of hypertension (headache, stiff neck, sweating, nausea, vomiting), and initiate medical treatment immediately.

• Monitor liver function; discontinue drug at first sign of hepatic dysfunction or jaundice.

• Discontinue drug and monitor BP carefully if patient reports unusual or severe headache.

• Provide phentolamine or another adrenergic blocking drug on standby in case hypertensive crisis occurs.

• Provide diet that is low in tyramine-containing foods.

Drug-Specific Patient Education

• Review the target symptoms that the drug potentially treats: depression.

• Review the dosing schedule until patient demonstrates a clear understanding of the regimen.

• Review the most common side effects: dizziness, weakness or fainting when arising from a horizontal or sitting position, drowsiness, blurred vision, nausea, vomiting, loss of appetite, nightmares, confusion, inability to concentrate, emotional changes, changes in sexual function.

• Review the side effects patient should report promptly: headache, skin rash, darkening of the urine, pale stools, yellowing of the eyes or skin, fever, chills, sore throat, or any other unusual symptoms.

• Caution patient to avoid the ingestion of tyramine-containing foods or beverages while on this drug and for 10 d after the drug is discontinued.

• Caution patient not to discontinue drug abruptly as serious side effects could occur.

• Caution patient to avoid the use of alcohol and sleep-inducing or OTC drugs.

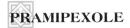

PRAMIPEXOLE

Mirapex

PREGNANCY CATEGORY C

Drug Classification: *Type:* antiparkinsonian; *Class:* nonergot dopamine agonist.

Mechanisms of Action

Stimulates dopamine receptors

in the striatum, leading to decrease in parkinsonism symptoms thought to be related to low dopamine levels.

Indications

Treatment of the signs and symptoms of idiopathic Parkinson's disease.

Contraindications/Cautions

Contraindications: • hypersensitivity to pramipexole.

Use cautiously with: • symptomatic hypotension • impaired renal function • pregnancy • lactation.

Dosage

Adult: Increase dosage gradually from a starting dose of 0.125 mg PO tid; week 2: 0.25 mg PO tid; week 3: 0.5 mg PO tid; week 4: 0.75 mg PO tid; week 5: 1 mg PO tid; week 6: 1.25 mg PO tid; week 7: 1.5 mg PO tid. If used in combination with levodopa, consider a reduction of dose. *Impaired Renal Function:* creatinine clearance (Ccr) >60 mg/dl, 0.125 mg PO tid starting dose to a maximum of 1.5 mg PO tid; Ccr 35–59 mg/dl, 0.125 mg PO bid starting dose to a maximum of 1.5 mg PO bid; Ccr 15–34 mg/dl, 0.125 mg PO qd starting dose to a maximum of 1.5 mg PO qd.

Pediatric Adolescent: Safety and efficacy not established.

Dosage Forms: Tablets: 0.125, 0.25, 1, 1.5 mg.

Blood Levels: Clinical significance is not established.

Pharmacokinetics

Absorption: rapid from the GI tract. *Distribution:* crosses blood–brain barrier, crosses placenta, may pass into breast milk. *Metabolism:* hepatic; $T_{1/2}$: 8 h. *Peak levels:* 2 h. *Excretion:* urine.

Adverse Effects

GI: Nausea, constipation, anorexia, dysphagia.

CNS: Headache, dizziness, insomnia, somnolence, hallucinations, confusion, amnesia.

CV: Orthostatic hypotension, hypertension, arrhythmia, palpitations, hypotension, tachycardia.

OTHER: Peripheral edema, decreased weight, asthenia, fever.

Clinically Important Drug–Drug Interactions

⇅ Increased levodopa levels and effects if combined.
⇅ Increased pramipexole levels when combined with cimetidine, ranitidine, diltiazem, truamterene, verapamil, quinidine, quinine.
⇅ Decreased effectiveness of pramipexole if taken in combination with dopamine antagonists.

Nursing Considerations

Assessment
• Assess for any of the conditions listed in "Contraindications/Cautions" above.
• Assess for ETOH or drug use/abuse and for concomitant prescribed and/or OTC medication.
• Complete physical exam: vital signs, weight, reflexes, affect, renal function.

Drug-Specific Patient Education
• Review the target symptoms that the drug potentially treats: tremor, drooling, shuffle, lack of coordination.
• Review the dosing schedule until patient demonstrates a clear understanding of the regimen: Take this drug three times a day, with breakfast and lunch. Continue to take your levodopa/carbidopa if prescribed. The dosage of the levodopa may need to be decreased after a few days of therapy. The dosage of pramipexole will be slowly increased over a 7-wk period. Write down dose and follow this pattern.
• Review the most common side effects: dizziness, lightheadedness, insomnia, nausea, edema, weight loss, hypotension.
• Review the side effects patient should report promptly: nausea, severe edema, sweating, hallucinations.

• Caution patient not to discontinue drug without consulting nurse or physician as serious side effects could occur; the drug should be tapered over at least a week.
• Caution patient to avoid the use of alcohol and sedative or OTC drugs.

PROCHLOR-PERAZINE

••••••••••••••••••••••••••••

Rectal suppositories: Compazine
   Prochlorperazine edisylate

Oral syrup, injection: Compazine
   Prochlorperazine maleate

Oral tablets and sustained-release capsules: Compazine, PMS-Prochlorperazine (CAN), Stemetil (CAN)

PREGNANCY CATEGORY C

Drug Classification: *Type:* antipsychotic, antiemetic, antianxiety; *Class:* dopaminergic blocking drug; *Subclass:* phenothiazine (piperazine).

Mechanisms of Action
Antipsychotic drugs block postsynaptic dopamine receptors in the brain, but this may not be necessary and sufficient for antipsychotic activity. Depresses the reticular activating

system, including those parts of the brain involved with wakefulness and emesis. Anticholinergic, antihistaminic (H1), and alpha-adrenergic blocking activity may also contribute to some of its therapeutic (and adverse) actions. Mechanism of action not fully understood.

Indications

Management of manifestations of psychotic disorders.

Short-term treatment of nonpsychotic anxiety (not drug of choice).

Contraindications/Cautions

Contraindications: • coma or severe CNS depression • bone marrow depression • blood dyscrasia • circulatory collapse • subcortical brain damage • Parkinson's disease • liver damage • cerebral arteriosclerosis • coronary disease • severe hypotension or hypertension.

Use cautiously with: • respiratory disorders • glaucoma • prostatic hypertrophy • epilepsy or history of epilepsy • breast cancer (elevations in prolactin may stimulate a prolactin-dependent tumor) • thyrotoxicosis • peptic ulcer • decreased renal function • myelography within previous 24 h or scheduled within 48 h • exposure to heat or phosphorus insecticides • pregnancy • lactation • children under 12 y of age, especially those with chicken pox • CNS infections.

Dosage

Adult: Initially 5–10 mg PO tid or qid. Gradually increase dosage every 2–3 d as necessary up to 50–75 mg/d for mild or moderate disturbances, 100–150 mg/d for more severe disturbances. For immediate control of severely disturbed adults, 10–20 mg IM repeated q 2–4 h (every hour for resistant cases); switch to oral therapy as soon as possible.

Pediatric: Generally not recommended for children under 20 lb. (9.1 kg) or 2 y of age; do not use in pediatric surgery. *2–12 y:* 2.5 mg PO or rectally bid–tid. Do not give more than 10 mg on the first day. Increase dosage according to patient response; total daily dose usually does not exceed 20 mg (children 2–5 y) or 25 mg (children 6–12 y). *<12 y:* 0.13 mg/kg by deep IM injection. Switch oral dosage as soon possible (usually after 1 dose).

Dosage Forms: Tablets: 5, 10, 25 mg; Spansules: 10, 15, 30 mg; Suppositories: 2.5, 5, 25 mg; Syrup: 5 mg/5 ml; Injection: 5 mg/ml.

Pharmacokinetics

Absorption: rapidly from the GI tract, rectal mucosa, muscle. *Distribution:* highly protein-bound; widely distributed; crosses placenta and passes into breast milk. *Metabolism:* hepatic; T_{1_2}: unknown. *Duration:* 3–4 h. *Elimination:* urine.

Adverse Effects

CNS: Drowsiness, insomnia, vertigo, headache, weakness, tremor, ataxia, slurring, cerebral edema, seizures, exacerbation of psychotic symptoms, extrapyramidal syndromes; pseudoparkinsonism; dystonias; akathisia, tardive dyskinesias, potentially irreversible; neuroleptic malignant syndrome.

EYE: Glaucoma, photophobia, blurred vision, miosis, mydriasis, deposits in the cornea and lens (opacities), pigmentary retinopathy.

HEMATOLOGIC: Eosinophilia, leukopenia, leukocytosis, anemia; aplastic anemia; hemolytic anemia; thrombocytopenic or nonthrombocytopenic purpura; pancytopenia.

CV: Hypotension, orthostatic hypotension, hypertension, tachycardia, bradycardia, cardiac arrest, CHF, cardiomegaly, refractory arrhythmias (some fatal), pulmonary edema.

RESPIRATORY: Bronchospasm, laryngospasm, dyspnea; suppression of cough reflex and potential for aspiration.

HYPERSENSITIVITY: Jaundice, urticaria, angioneurotic edema, laryngeal edema, photosensitivity, eczema, asthma, anaphylactoid reactions, exfoliative dermatitis.

ENDOCRINE: Lactation, breast engorgement in females, galactorrhea; syndrome of inappropriate ADH secretion (SIADH); amenorrhea, menstrual irregularities; gynecomastia in males; changes in libido; hyperglycemia or hypoglycemia; glycosuria; hyponatremia; pituitary tumor with hyperprolactinemia; inhibition of ovulation, infertility, pseudopregnancy; reduced urinary levels of gonadotropins, estrogens, progestins.

AUTONOMIC: Dry mouth, salivation, nasal congestion, nausea, vomiting, anorexia, fever, pallor, flushed facies, sweating, constipation, paralytic ileus, urinary retention, incontinence, polyuria, enuresis, priapism, ejaculation inhibition, male impotence.

OTHER: Urine discolored pink to red-brown.

Clinically Important Drug–Drug Interactions

⇥ Additive CNS depression with alcohol.

⇇ Additive anticholinergic effects and possibly decreased antipsychotic efficacy with anticholinergic drugs.

⇇ Increased likelihood of seizures with metrizamide.

⇇ Increased chance of severe neuromuscular excitation and hypotension if given to patients receiving barbiturate anesthetics (methohexital, thiamylal, phenobarbital, thiopental).

⇇ Decreased antihypertensive effect of guanethidine when taken concurrently.

Nursing Considerations

Assessment

• Assess for any conditions listed under "Contraindications/Cautions" above.

• Assess for any history of drug abuse or dependence, current use of prescribed or OTC medications.

• Complete physical exam: vital signs, orthostatic BP, intraocular pressure, CBC, urinalysis; thyroid, liver, and kidney function tests.

• Assess for consistent use of brand names of oral preparations; bioavailability differences have been documented for different brands.

• Arrange for discontinuation of drug if serum creatinine or BUN become abnormal or if WBC count is depressed.

• Assess elderly patients for dehydration and institute remedial measures promptly if it occurs; sedation and decreased sensation of thirst related to CNS effects of drug can lead to severe dehydration.

Drug-Specific Patient Education

• Review the target symptoms that the drug potentially treats: manifestations of psychoses.

• Review the dosing schedule until patient demonstrates a clear understanding of drug regimen.

• Review the most common side effects: sensitivity to the sun, dizziness, drowsiness, vision changes, dehydration, increased heat intolerance, pink or reddish brown urine.

• Review the side effects patient should report promptly: sore throat, fever, unusual bleeding or bruising, rash, weakness, tremors, impaired vision, dark-colored urine, pale stools, yellowing of the skin or eyes.

• Caution patient to avoid sun exposure; use of a sunscreen and protective clothing is advised.

• Caution patient to maintain fluid intake and use precautions against heatstroke in hot weather.

• Caution patient to avoid alcohol and sleep-inducing or OTC medications.

PROPRANOLOL HYDROCHLORIDE

••••••••••••••••••••••••

Apo-Propranolol (CAN), Inderal, Novopranol (CAN), PMS-Propranolol (CAN), Propranolol Intensol

PREGNANCY CATEGORY C

Drug Classification: *Type:* antianginal, antiarrhythmic, antihypertensive; *Class:* beta-adrenergic blocker; *Subclass:* nonselective beta-blocker.

Mechanisms of Action

Competitively blocks beta-adrenergic receptors in the heart and juxtaglomerular apparatus, decreasing the influence of the sympathetic nervous system on these tissues and decreasing the excitability of the heart, decreasing cardiac work load and oxygen consumption, decreasing the release of renin, and lowering blood pressure; has membrane-stabilizing (local anesthetic) effects that contribute to its antiarrhythmic action. Acts in the CNS to reduce sympathetic outflow and vasoconstrictor tone. Blocks the signs and symptoms of a stress reaction.

Indications

Management of acute situational stress reaction (stage fright). Treatment of essential tremor, familial or hereditary. *Unlabeled uses:* Treatment of schizophrenia, tardive dyskinesia, acute panic symptoms, Parkinsonian tremors, alcohol withdrawal symptoms, aggressive behavior, antipsychotic-induced akathisia.

Contraindications/Cautions

Contraindications: • allergy to beta blocking agents • sinus bradycardia • 2nd or 3rd degree heart block • cardiogenic shock • CHF • bronchial asthma • bronchospasm • COPD • pregnancy • lactation.
  Use cautiously with: • hypoglycemia and diabetes • thyrotoxicosis • hepatic dysfunction.

Dosage

Adult: *Essential tremor:* 40 mg bid; usual maintenance dose 120 mg/d. *Aggressive behavior:* 80–300 mg PO qd. *Antipsychotic induced akathisia:* 20–80 mg PO qd. *Parkinsonian tremors:* 160 mg PO qd. *Situational anxiety:* 40 mg, timing based on the usual onset of action. *Schizophrenia:* 300–5000 mg PO qd. *Acute panic symptoms:* 40–320 mg PO qd. *Anxiety:* 80–320 mg PO qd.

Pediatric Adolescent: Safety and efficacy not established.

Dosage Forms: Tablets: 10, 20, 40, 60, 80, 90 mg; Sustained release capsules: 60, 80, 120, 160 mg; Oral solution: 4 mg/ml, 8 mg/ml; Concentrated oral solution: 80 mg/ml.

Pharmacokinetics

Absorption: rapidly from the GI tract. *Distribution:* highly lipid soluble; highly protein-bound; widely distributed; crosses placenta and passes into breast milk. *Metabolism:* hepatic; $T_{1/2}$: 3–5 h. *Peak levels:* 60–90 min. *Duration:* 4–6 h. *Elimination:* urine.

Adverse Effects

CV: Bradycardia, CHF, cardiac arrhythmias, sinoatrial or AV nodal block, tachycardia, peripheral vascular insufficiency, claudication, CVA, pulmonary edema, hypotension, dizziness, vertigo, tinnitus, fatigue, emotional depression, paresthesias, sleep disturbances, hallucinations, disorientation, memory loss, slurred speech.

RESPIRATORY: Bronchospasm, dyspnea, cough, bronchial obstruction, nasal stuffiness, rhinitis, pharyngitis (less likely than with propranolol).

GI: Gastric pain, flatulence, constipation, diarrhea, nausea, vomiting, anorexia, ischemic colitis, renal and mesenteric arterial thrombosis, retroperitoneal fibrosis, hepatomegaly, acute pancreatitis.

GU: Impotence, decreased libido, Peyronie's disease, dysuria, nocturia, frequent urination.

SKELETAL: Joint pain, arthralgia, muscle cramp.

SKIN: Rash, pruritus, sweating, dry skin.

EYES: Eye irritation, dry eyes, conjunctivitis, blurred vision.

ALLERGIC REACTIONS: Pharyngitis, erythematous rash, fever, sore throat, laryngospasm, respiratory distress.

OTHER: Decreased exercise tolerance, development of antinuclear antibodies (ANA), hyperglycemia or hypoglycemia, elevated serum transaminase, alkaline phosphatase, and LDH.

Clinically Important Drug–Drug Interactions

⸭ Increased effects of propranolol with verapamil; decreased effects of propranolol with indomethacin, ibuprofen, piroxicam, sulindac, barbiturates.
⸭ Prolonged hypoglycemic effects of insulin if taken concurrently with propranolol.
⸭ Peripheral ischemia possible if propranolol combined with ergot alkaloids.
⸭ Initial hypertensive episode followed by bradycardia if

taken concurrently with epinephrine.

⚁ Increased "first-dose response" to prazosin when taken concurrently with propranolol.

⚁ Increased serum levels and toxic effects if taken concurrently with lidocaine, cimetidine.

⚁ Increased serum levels of both propranolol and phenothiazines, hydralazine if the two drugs are taken concurrently.

⚁ Paradoxical hypertension when clonidine is given with beta-blockers; increased rebound hypertension when clonidine is discontinued in patients on beta-blockers.

⚁ Decreased serum levels and therapeutic effects if propranolol is taken with methimazole, propylthiouracil.

⚁ Decreased bronchodilator effects of theophyllines taken with propranolol.

⚁ Decreased antihypertensive effects of propranolol if taken concurrently with NSAIDs (i.e., ibuprofen, indomethacin, piroxicam, sulindac), rifampin.

Nursing Considerations

Assessment
• Assess for any conditions listed under "Contraindications/Cautions" above.

• Assess for history of drug use or dependence, current use of prescribed or OTC medications.

• Complete physical exam: vital signs, kidney and thyroid function, blood and urine glucose.

Drug-Specific Patient Education
• Review the target symptoms that the drug potentially treats: signs and symptoms of anxiety, tremors, cognitive function, aggressive behavior.

• Review the dosing schedule until patient demonstrates a clear understanding of drug regimen.

• Review the most common side effects: dizziness, lightheadedness, loss of appetite, nightmares, depression, sexual impotence, nausea.

• Review the side effects patient should report promptly: difficulty breathing, night cough, swelling of extremities, slow pulse, confusion, depression, rash, fever, sore throat.

• Caution patient not to stop taking drug abruptly as serious side effects could occur; must be tapered over time.

• Caution diabetic patients that signs and symptoms of hypo- and hyperglycemic reactions may be blocked.

• Caution patient to avoid alcohol and sleep-inducing or OTC medications.

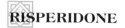

RISPERIDONE

••••••••••••••••••••••••••

Risperdal

PREGNANCY CATEGORY C

Drug Classification: *Type:* antipsychotic drug; *Class:* benzisoxazole.

Mechanisms of Action
Blocks dopamine and serotonin receptors in the brain, depresses the reticular activating system. Anticholinergic, antihistaminic, and alpha-adrenergic blocking activity may contribute to some of its therapeutic and adverse actions; mechanism of action not fully understood.

Indications
Management of the manifestations of psychotic disorders.
Unlabeled use: Relief of symptoms of PMS (premenstrual syndrome).

Contraindications/Cautions
Contraindications: • allergy to risperidone, lactation.
  Use cautiously with:
• cardiovascular disease
• pregnancy • renal or hepatic impairment • hypotension.

Dosage
Adult: Initially 1 mg PO bid; then gradually continue to increase with daily dosage increments of 1 mg/d on the second and third days to a target dose of 3 mg PO bid by the third day. *Reinitiation of treatment:* Follow initial dosage guidelines, using extreme care due to increased risk of severe adverse effects with reexposure. *Switching from other antipsychotics:* Minimize the overlap period and discontinue other antipsychotic before beginning risperidone therapy.

Pediatric Adolescent: Safety and efficacy not established.

Geriatric or Renal/Hepatic Impaired: Initial dose of 0.5 mg PO bid; monitor patient for adverse effects and response.

Dosage Forms: Tablets: 1, 2, 3, 4 mg.

Pharmacokinetics
Absorption: rapidly from the GI tract. *Distribution:* plasma protein-bound; crosses placenta and passes into breast milk. *Metabolism:* hepatic; $T_{1/2}$: 20 h. *Steady state:* 6–9 d. *Elimination:* urine and feces.

Adverse Effects
CNS: Insomnia, anxiety, agitation, headache, somnolence, aggression. dizziness, tardive dyskinesias.
GI: Nausea, vomiting, constipation, abdominal discomfort, dry mouth, increased saliva.

RESPIRATORY: Rhinitis, coughing, sinusitis, pharyngitis, dyspnea.

DERMATOLOGIC: Rash, dry skin, seborrhea, photosensitivity.

CV: Orthostatic hypotension, arrhythmias.

OTHER: Chest pain, arthralgia, back pain, fever, Neuroleptic Malignant Syndrome (NMS).

Clinically Important Drug–Drug Interactions

⚮ Increased therapeutic and toxic effects of risperidone if taken with clozapine.

⚮ Decreased therapeutic effect of risperidone if taken with carbamazepine.

⚮ Decreased effectiveness of levodopa if taken concurrently.

Nursing Considerations

Assessment

• Assess for conditions listed under "Contraindications/Cautions" above.

• Assess for history of alcohol or drug dependence or abuse, current use of prescribed or OTC medications.

• Complete physical exam: vital signs, orthostatic BP, reflexes, orientation, CBC, urinalysis, liver and kidney function tests.

Drug-Specific Patient Education

• Review the target symptoms that the drug potentially treats: relief of manifestations of psychosis.

• Review the dosing schedule until patient demonstrates clear understanding of regimen.

• Review the most common side effects: drowsiness, dizziness, sedation, seizures; dizziness, faintness on arising; increased salivation; constipation; sensitivity to the sun.

• Review the side effects patient should report promptly: lethargy, weakness, fever, sore throat, malaise, mouth ulcers, palpitations.

• Caution patient not to discontinue drug abruptly as serious side effects could occur.

• Caution patient to avoid pregnancy; use of barrier contraceptives is advised.

• Caution patient to avoid the use of alcohol and sleep-inducing or OTC medications.

SERTRALINE HYDROCHLORIDE

Zoloft

PREGNANCY CATEGORY B

Drug Classification: *Type:* specific serotonin reuptake inhibitor (SSRI); antidepressant.

Mechanisms of Action

Antidepressant activity associated with presynaptic reuptake of serotonin; no significant effects on norepinephrine, dopamine, or on adrenergic, histaminergic, muscarinic, and serotonergic receptors.

Indications

Treatment of depression, dysthymia, social phobia, obsessive-compulsive disorder, panic, premenstrual dysphoric disorder.

Contraindications/Cautions

Contraindications: • hypersensitivity to sertraline • pregnancy • lactation

Use cautiously with:
• impaired hepatic or renal function • may precipitate mania.

Dosage

Adult: 25–200 mg/d. May be given qd, usually in a.m. Earliest onset of action within 2–5 d. Consider drug trial a failure if patient has been on maximum recommended dose for 4–6 wk without response.

Pediatric Adolescent: Start at one-half the adult dose and increase slowly and cautiously.

Geriatric: Start at one-half the adult dose and increase slowly and cautiously.

Dosage Forms: Tablets: 50, 100 mg.

Pharmacokinetics

Absorption: from the GI tract; reaches peak plasma levels in 6–8 h. *Distribution:* tightly bound to plasma protein; crosses placenta, enters breast milk. *Metabolism:* hepatic; T_{1_2}: 26 h. *Steady state:* 7 d. *Elimination:* urine and feces.

Adverse Effects

CNS: Headaches, nervousness, insomnia, drowsiness, anxiety, tremor, dizziness, fatigue, sedation, sensation disturbance, decreased libido, light-headedness, decreased concentration.

GI: Nausea, diarrhea, dry mouth, anorexia, dyspepsia, constipation, abdominal pain, vomiting, taste change, flatulence, gastroenteritis.

SKIN: Excessive sweating, rash, pruritus.

BODY AS A WHOLE: Asthenia, chest and limb pain, fever.

RESPIRATORY: Rhinitis, flu-like syndrome, pharyngitis, dyspnea.

CV: Hot flashes, palpitations.

MUSCULOSKELETAL: Back, joint, and muscle pain.

GU: Painful menstruation, sexual dysfunction.

SPECIAL SENSES: Visual disturbance.

Clinically Important Drug–Drug Interactions

⌐ *Note:* The use of other drugs tightly bound to protein (e.g., warfarin, digitoxin) may cause a shift in plasma concentrations, potentially resulting in adverse effects; prothrombin time should be carefully monitored when given with sertraline.

⌐ Toxic reactions or serotonin syndrome may occur with MAOIs or L-tryptophan.

⌐ May decrease clearance of tolbutamide.

Nursing Considerations

Assessment

• Assess for any of the conditions listed in "Contraindications/Cautions" above.

• Assess for concurrent prescription, OTC, or illegal drug or ETOH use/abuse; risk of suicide. Limit potentially suicidal patients' access to drug.

• Complete physical, vital signs, weight; CBC with differential; liver and thyroid function tests; BUN; creatinine; ECG if >40 y.

Drug-Specific Patient Education

• Review target symptoms that drug potentially treats: disruptions in sleep, appetite, concentration, energy, mood; anhedonia; interest; motivation; initiative; suicidal idea-

tion, panic, obsessions, compulsions.

• Review dosing schedule until patient demonstrates a clear understanding of regimen.

• Discuss expected lag period (3–4 wk) before full therapeutic effects can be anticipated.

• Review most common side effects (agitation, anxiety, dizziness, insomnia, nausea, sweating, anorexia, diarrhea, tremor) and encourage patient to report any side effects promptly.

• Educate patient about contraception during drug use.

• Caution patient about concurrent ETOH and drug use.

THIORIDAZINE HYDROCHLORIDE

Apo-Thioridazine (CAN), Mellaril

PREGNANCY CATEGORY C

Drug Classification: *Type:* dopamine receptor antagonist; also called antipsychotic, neuroleptic, or major tranquilizer; *Class:* phenothiazine; *Subclass:* piperidine.

Mechanisms of Action

Postsynaptic antagonism of dopamine receptors, primarily D2 (antipsychotic efficacy is thought to be mediated by these actions). Blockade of muscarinic cholinergic, noradrenergic, and histaminergic receptors (some undesirable side effects are thought to be mediated by these actions).

Indications

Short- and long-term management of idiopathic psychoses including schizophrenia, schizophreniform disorder, schizoaffective disorder, delusional disorder, brief psychotic disorder, mania with psychosis, and major depressive disorder with psychotic features.

Secondary psychoses associated with a general medical condition or substance-related disorder.

Acute deliria and organic psychoses.

Severe anxiety, agitation or violent behavior.

Severe behavioral problems in children marked by combativeness and/or explosive hyperexcitability and in the short-term treatment of hyperactive children who show excessive motor activity.

Movement disorder of Huntington's disease.

Motor and vocal tics of Tourette's Syndrome.

Brief use for episodes of severe dyscontrol or apparent psychosis in some personality disorders.

Control of nausea, vomiting, and intractable hiccups.

Depression with marked anxiety or agitation.

Contraindications/Cautions

Contraindications: • allergy to thioridazine • comatose or severely depressed states • presence of large amounts of CNS depressants (alcohol, barbiturates, narcotics, etc.) • bone marrow depression • blood dyscrasias • circulatory collapse • subcortical brain damage • Parkinson's disease • liver damage • cerebral or coronary arteriosclerosis • CV disease • severe hypotension or hypertension • respiratory disorders • glaucoma • history of epilepsy or seizures • peptic ulcer or history of peptic ulcer • decreased renal function • urinary retention, ureteral or urethral spasm • prostate hypertrophy • breast cancer • thyrotoxicosis • myelography within 24 h or scheduled within 48 h • pregnancy • lactation • exposure to heat, organophosphorous insecticides, or atropine or related drugs • children with chickenpox • CNS infections • if signs and symptoms of tardive dyskinesia appear, drug discontinuation should be considered • history of neuroleptic malignant syndrome.

Dosage

Adult: Patients may respond to widely different dosages of antipsychotics. Therefore, there is no set dosage for any given antipsychotic drug. Usual range for acute use (oral): 200–600 mg/d. Usual range for maintenance use (oral): 100–600 mg/d. Can be administered once a day.

Pediatric Adolescent: Generally not used in children <2 y; 0.5–3 mg/kg/d.

Geriatric: Start dosage at one-fourth to one-third that given in younger adults and increase more gradually.

Dosage Forms: Tablets: 10, 25, 50, 100, 150, 200 mg; Liquid concentrate: 30 mg/ml; Elixir: 25 mg/5ml.

Pharmacokinetics

Absorption: (oral) adequate but variable; food or antacids may decrease absorption; liquid preparations are absorbed more rapidly and reliably than tablets; onset of action 3–60 min; peak level: 2–4 h. *Distribution:* highly protein bound (85–90%) and lipophilic; readily crosses the blood–brain barrier, placenta, and enters breast milk; concentrations in the brain appear to be greater than those in blood; not removed efficiently by dialysis. *Metabolism:* hepatic.

Elimination: urine. The elimination half-life of most antipsychotic drugs is 18–40 h; plasma levels may vary among individuals by 10- to 20-fold.

Adverse Effects

CNS: Drowsiness, insomnia, vertigo, headache, weakness, tremors, ataxia, slurring of speech, cerebral edema, seizures, exacerbation of psychotic symptoms, extrapyramidal syndromes (EPS), neuroleptic malignant syndrome, tardive dyskinesia, pseudo-parkinsonism, akathisia (see descriptions of symptoms under "Implementation" below).

GI: Dry mouth, salivation, nausea, vomiting, anorexia, constipation, paralytic ileus.

CV: Hypotension, orthostatic hypotension, hypertension, tachycardia, bradycardia, cardiac arrest, CHF, cardiomegaly, refractory arrhythmias, dysrhythmias, pulmonary edema.

RESPIRATORY: Bronchospasm, laryngospasm, dyspnea, suppression of cough reflex, and potential aspiration.

HEMATOLOGIC: Eosinophilia, leukopenia, leukocytosis, anemia, aplastic anemia, hemolytic anemia, thrombocytopenic or nonthrombocytopenic purpura, pancytopenia, elevated serum cholesterol.

GU: Urinary retention,

polyuria, incontinence, priapism, ejaculation inhibition, male impotence, urine discolored pink to red-brown.

EENT: Nasal congestion, glaucoma, photophobia, blurred vision, miosis, mydriasis, deposits in the cornea and lens, pigmentary retinopathy.

HYPERSENSITIVITY: Jaundice, urticaria, angioneurotic edema, laryngeal edema, photosensitivity, eczema, asthma, anaphylactoid reactions, exfoliative dermatitis, contact dermatitis.

ENDOCRINE: Lactation, breast engorgement in females, galactorrhea, syndrome of inappropriate ADH secretion, amenorrhea, menstrual irregularities, gynecomastia, changes in libido, hyperglycemia, inhibition of ovulation, infertility, pseudopregnancy, reduced urinary levels of gonadotropins, estrogens, and progestins.

OTHER: Fever, heat stroke, pallor, flushed facies, sweating.

Clinically Important Drug–Drug Interactions

⊞ Additive anticholinergic effects and possibly decreased antipsychotic efficacy with anticholinergic drugs.
⊞ Additive CNS depression and hypotension with barbiturates, alcohol, meperidine.
⊞ Additive effects of both drugs with beta-blockers.
⊞ Increased risk of tachycardia, hypotension with epinephrine, norepinephrine.
⊞ Increased risk of seizure with metrizamide.
⊞ Decreased hypotensive effect with guanethidine.
⊞ Because of displacement and competition for protein-binding sites, concomitant treatment with other highly protein-bound medications (e.g., warfarin, digoxin) could alter concentrations of both drugs.
⊞ Decreased effect of oral anticoagulants.
⊞ Possible increase in phenytoin levels.

Lab Test Interference

• False-positive pregnancy tests (less likely if serum test is used).
• Increase in protein-bound iodine not attributable to an increase in thyroxine.
• Blood levels of antipsychotics have not correlated well with clinical response, and serum levels are probably more misleading than useful.

Nursing Considerations

Assessment

• Assess for any of the conditions listed under "Contraindications/Cautions" above.
• Assess for alcohol and drug use/abuse and for concomitant use of prescription and/or OTC medications.
• Assess for risk of suicidality.

• Complete physical exam: vital signs including orthostatic BP, ECG, CBC with differential, thyroid and liver function, BUN, creatinine.

Implementation

• Bioavailability differs between brand names of oral forms.

• Dilute liquid concentrate just before administration in 60 ml or more of fruit juice, milk, simple syrup, orange syrup, carbonated beverage, coffee, tea, water, or semisolid foods.

• Protect liquid concentrate from light.

• Be alert to potential for aspiration because of suppressed cough reflex.

• Monitor for dehydration, renal or liver abnormalities, depressed WBC, symptoms of infection. Promptly report to prescriber and institute remedial measures.

• Monitor for extrapyramidal side effects (involuntary dystonic muscular movements of the neck, jaw, tongue, or entire body; swallowing difficulties; oculogyric crisis); Parkinsonism (muscle stiffness; cogwheel rigidity; shuffling gait, stooped posture, drooling, coarse tremor, "rabbit syndrome," masklike facies, bradykinesia, akinesia); akathisia (subjective feeling of muscular discomfort that can cause agitation, restlessness, pacing, rocking, continually changing posture, and dysphoria).

• Monitor for symptoms of neuroleptic malignant syndrome: muscle rigidity; altered mental status; evidence of autonomic instability (e.g., irregular pulse or blood pressure, tachycardia, cardiac dysrhythmias); hyperpyrexia, sweating; increased WBC, blood creatinine phosphokinase, liver enzymes, myoglobin; mutism, obtundation, agitation.

• Monitor for symptoms of tardive dyskinesia (abnormal, involuntary, irregular, choreoathetoid movements of muscles of the head, limbs, and trunk; darting, twisting, and protruding movements of the tongue; chewing and lateral jaw movements; lip puckering; facial grimacing; finger movements and hand clenching; torticollis, retrocollis, trunk twisting, pelvic thrusting).

• Taper drug gradually after high-dose therapy due to possible gastritis, nausea, dizziness, headache, tachycardia, insomnia after abrupt withdrawal.

Drug-Specific Patient Education

• Review target symptoms that drug potentially treats: auditory, visual, olfactory, tactile hallucinations; delusions; paranoia; disorders of thought and speech; psychotic agitation; insomnia.

• Review dosing schedule until patient demonstrates a clear understanding of regimen. Caution patient against changing dosage or discontinuation without consulting prescriber.

• Caution patient against concurrent alcohol or drug use.

• Discuss expected lag period (6 wk or more) before full therapeutic effects appear.

• Review most common side effects (drowsiness, insomnia, dry mouth, constipation, dizziness from hypotension, urinary hesitancy or retention, photosensitivity, blurred vision, urticaria, EPS, Parkinsonism, akathisia), and encourage patient to report any side effects promptly.

• If possible, give the patient full information about the risk of tardive dyskinesia and possible irreversibility. (The decision whether to inform patients and/or their guardians must take into account the clinical circumstances and the competency of the patient to understand the information provided.)

• Educate patient about possibly life-threatening blood dyscrasias and instruct patient to report fever, chills, sore throat, unusual bleeding or bruising, or rash and to discontinue medication immediately (most likely between 4th and 10th weeks of treatment).

• Caution patient about risk of dehydration or heat stroke, increased sensitivity to sunburn, and warn against over exercising in a hot climate.

THIOTHIXENE HYDROCHLORIDE

Navane

PREGNANCY CATEGORY C

Drug Classification: *Type:* dopamine receptor antagonist; also called antipsychotic, neuroleptic, or major tranquilizer; *Class:* thioxanthene; *Subclass:* piperazine.

Mechanisms of Action

Postsynaptic antagonism of dopamine receptors, primarily D2 (antipsychotic efficacy is thought to be mediated by these actions). Blockade of muscarinic cholinergic, noradrenergic, and histaminergic receptors (some undesirable side effects are thought to be mediated by these actions).

Indications

Short- and long-term management of idiopathic psychoses including schizophrenia, schizophreniform disorder, schizoaffective disorder, delusional disorder, brief psychotic disorder, mania with psychosis, and major depressive disorder with psychotic features.

Secondary psychoses associated with a general medical condition or substance-related disorder.

Acute deliria and organic psychoses.

Severe agitation or violent behavior.

Severe behavioral problems in children marked by combativeness and/or explosive hyperexcitability and in the short-term treatment of hyperactive children who show excessive motor activity.

Movement disorder of Huntington's disease.

Motor and vocal tics of Tourette's Syndrome.

Brief use for episodes of severe dyscontrol or apparent psychosis in some personality disorders.

Control of nausea, vomiting, and intractable hiccups.

Contraindications/Cautions

Contraindications: • allergy to thiothixene • comatose or severely depressed states • presence of large amounts of CNS depressants (alcohol, barbiturates, narcotics, etc.) • bone marrow depression • blood dyscrasias • circulatory collapse • subcortical brain damage • Parkinson's disease • liver damage • cerebral or coronary arteriosclerosis • CV disease • severe hypotension or hypertension • respiratory disorders • glaucoma • history of epilepsy or seizures • peptic ulcer or history of peptic ulcer • decreased renal function • urinary retention, ureteral or urethral spasm • prostate hypertrophy • breast cancer • thyrotoxicosis • myelography within 24 h or scheduled within 48 h • pregnancy • lactation • exposure to heat, organophosphorous insecticides, or atropine or related drugs • children with chickenpox • CNS infections • if signs and symptoms of tardive dyskinesia appear, drug discontinuation should be considered • history of neuroleptic malignant syndrome.

Dosage

Adult: Patients may respond to widely different dosages of antipsychotics. Therefore, there is no set dosage for any given antipsychotic drug. Usual range for acute use (oral): 6–30 mg/d. Usual range for maintenance use (oral): 5–25 mg/d. Can be administered once a day. IM: oral forms should be used whenever possible, but IM forms may be necessary for patients who exhibit violent behavior or for those who have high first-pass or presystemic metabolism of oral forms. Starting dose 2 mg IM; may repeat in 1 h; increase dosage gradually up to 30 mg/d (maximum). Switch to oral dosage as soon as patient is able or willing.

Pediatric Adolescent: Generally not used in children <12 y; >12 may start on lowest adult dose.

Geriatric: Start dosage at one-fourth to one-third that given in younger adults and increase more gradually.

Dosage Forms: Tablets: 11, 2, 5, 10, 20 mg; Liquid concentrate: 5 mg/ml; Injection: 2, 5 mg/ml.

Pharmacokinetics

Absorption: (oral) adequate but variable; food or antacids may decrease absorption; liquid preparations are absorbed more rapidly and reliably than tablets; onset of action 3–60 min; peak level: 2–4 h; IM rapidly and reliably absorbed; onset of action 15–20 min; peak: 30–60 min. *Distribution:* highly protein bound (85–90%) and lipophilic; readily crosses the blood–brain barrier, placenta, and enters breast milk; concentrations in the brain appear to be greater than those in blood; not removed efficiently by dialysis. *Metabolism:* hepatic. *Elimination:* urine. The elimination half-life of most antipsychotic drugs is 18–40 h; plasma levels may vary among individuals by 10- to 20-fold.

Adverse Effects

CNS: Drowsiness, insomnia, vertigo, headache, weakness, tremors, ataxia, slurring of speech, cerebral edema, seizures, exacerbation of psychotic symptoms, extrapyramidal syndromes (EPS), neuroleptic malignant syndrome, tardive dyskinesia, pseudo-parkinsonism, akathisia (see descriptions of symptoms under "Implementation" below).

GI: Dry mouth, salivation, nausea, vomiting, anorexia, constipation, paralytic ileus.

CV: Hypotension, orthostatic hypotension, hypertension, tachycardia, bradycardia, cardiac arrest, CHF, cardiomegaly, refractory arrhythmias, dysrhythmias, pulmonary edema.

RESPIRATORY: Bronchospasm, laryngospasm, dyspnea, suppression of cough reflex, and potential aspiration.

HEMATOLOGIC: Eosinophilia, leukopenia, leukocytosis, anemia, aplastic anemia, hemolytic anemia, thrombocytopenic or nonthrombocytopenic purpura, pancytopenia, elevated serum cholesterol.

GU: Urinary retention, polyuria, incontinence, priapism, ejaculation inhibition, male impotence, urine discolored pink to red-brown.

EENT: Nasal congestion, glaucoma, photophobia, blurred vision, miosis, mydriasis, deposits in the cornea and lens, pigmentary retinopathy.

HYPERSENSITIVITY: Jaundice, urticaria, angioneurotic edema, laryngeal edema, photosensitivity, eczema, asthma, anaphylactoid reactions, exfoliative dermatitis, contact dermatitis.

ENDOCRINE: Lactation, breast engorgement in females, galactorrhea, syndrome of inappropriate ADH secretion, amenorrhea, menstrual irregularities, gynecomastia, changes in libido, hyperglycemia, inhibition of ovulation, infertility, pseudopregnancy, reduced urinary levels of gonadotropins, estrogens, and progestins.

OTHER: Fever, heat stroke, pallor, flushed facies, sweating.

Clinically Important Drug–Drug Interactions

⌗ Additive anticholinergic effects and possibly decreased antipsychotic efficacy with anticholinergic drugs.
⌗ Additive CNS depression and hypotension with barbiturates, alcohol, meperidine.
⌗ Additive effects of both drugs with beta-blockers.
⌗ Increased risk of tachycardia, hypotension with epinephrine, norepinephrine.
⌗ Increased risk of seizure with metrizamide.
⌗ Decreased hypotension effect with guanethidine.
⌗ Because of displacement and competition for protein-binding sites, concomitant treatment with other highly protein-bound medications (e.g., warfarin, digoxin) could alter concentrations of both drugs.
⌗ Decreased effect of oral anticoagulants.
⌗ Possible increase in phenytoin levels.

Lab Test Interference

• False-positive pregnancy tests (less likely if serum test is used).
• Increase in protein-bound iodine, not attributable to an increase in thyroxine.
• Blood levels of antipsychotics have not correlated well with clinical response and serum levels are probably more misleading than useful.

Nursing Considerations

Assessment

• Assess for any of the conditions listed under "Contraindications/Cautions" above.
• Assess for alcohol and drug use/abuse and for concomitant use of prescription and/or OTC medications.
• Assess for risk of suicidality.

• Complete physical exam: vital signs including orthostatic BP, ECG, CBC with differential, thyroid and liver function, BUN, creatinine.

Implementation
• Bioavailability differs between brand names of oral forms.
• Dilute liquid concentrate just before administration in 60 ml or more of fruit juice, milk, simple syrup, orange syrup, carbonated beverage, coffee, tea, water, or semisolid foods.
• Protect liquid concentrate from light.
• Give IM injection slowly into upper outer-quadrant of buttock.
• Be alert to potential for aspiration because of suppressed cough reflex.
• Monitor for dehydration, renal or liver abnormalities, depressed WBC, symptoms of infection. Promptly report to prescriber and institute remedial measures.
• Monitor for extrapyramidal side effects (involuntary dystonic muscular movements of the neck, jaw, tongue, or entire body; swallowing difficulties; oculogyric crisis); Parkinsonism (muscle stiffness; cogwheel rigidity; shuffling gait, stooped posture, drooling, coarse tremor, "rabbit syndrome," masklike facies, bradykinesia, akinesia); akathisia (subjective feeling of muscular discomfort that can cause agitation, restlessness, pacing, rocking, continually changing posture, and dysphoria).
• Monitor for symptoms of Neuroleptic Malignant Syndrome: muscle rigidity; altered mental status; evidence of autonomic instability (e.g., irregular pulse or blood pressure, tachycardia, cardiac dysrhythmias); hyperpyrexia, sweating; increased WBC, blood creatinine phosphokinase, liver enzymes, myoglobin; mutism, obtundation, agitation.
• Monitor for symptoms of tardive dyskinesia (abnormal, involuntary, irregular, choreoathetoid movements of muscles of the head, limbs, and trunk; darting, twisting, and protruding movements of the tongue; chewing and lateral jaw movements; lip puckering; facial grimacing; finger movements and hand clenching; torticollis, retrocollis, trunk twisting, pelvic thrusting).
• Taper drug gradually after high-dose therapy due to possible gastritis, nausea, dizziness, headache, tachycardia, insomnia after abrupt withdrawal.

Drug-Specific Patient Education
• Review target symptoms that drug potentially treats: auditory, visual, olfactory, tactile hallucinations; delusions; paranoia; disorders of thought and speech; psychotic agitation; insomnia.

• Review dosing schedule until patient demonstrates a clear understanding of regimen. Caution patient against changing dosage or discontinuation without consulting prescriber.

• Caution patient against concurrent alcohol or drug use.

• Discuss expected lag period (6 wk or more) before full therapeutic effects appear.

• Review most common side effects (drowsiness, insomnia, dry mouth, constipation, dizziness from hypotension, urinary hesitancy or retention, photosensitivity, blurred vision, urticaria, EPS, Parkinsonism, akathisia) and encourage patient to report any side effects promptly.

• If possible, give the patient full information about the risk of tardive dyskinesia and possible irreversibility. (The decision whether to inform patients and/or their guardians must take into account the clinical circumstances and the competency of the patient to understand the information provided.)

• Educate patient about possibly life-threatening blood dyscrasias and instruct patient to report fever, chills, sore throat, unusual bleeding or bruising, or rash and to discontinue medication immediately (most likely between 4th and 10th weeks of treatment).

• Caution patient about risk of dehydration or heat stroke, increased risk of sunburn and warn against over exercising in a hot climate.

TRANYL-CYPROMINE SULFATE

Parnate

PREGNANCY CATEGORY C

Drug Classification: *Type:* antidepressant; *Class:* monoamine oxidase inhibitor (MAOI); *Subclass:* hydrazine derivative.

Mechanisms of Action

Irreversibly inhibits monoamine oxidase, an enzyme that breaks down biogenic amines such as epinephrine, norepinephrine, and serotonin, allowing these biogenic amines to accumulate in neuronal storage sites. According to the "biogenic amine hypothesis," this accumulation of amines is responsible for the clinical efficacy of MAOIs as antidepressants.

Indications

Treatment of adult outpatients with reactive depression; efficacy in endogenous depression has not been established. *Unlabeled use:* Treatment of bulimia having characteristics of atypical depression.

Contraindications/Cautions

Contraindications: • hypersensitivity to any MAOI • pheochromocytoma, CHF • history of liver disease or abnormal liver function tests • severe renal impairment • confirmed or suspected cerebrovascular defect • cardiovascular disease • hypertension • history of headache • myelography within previous 24 h or scheduled within 48 h • lactation.

Use cautiously with: • seizure disorders • hyperthyroidism • impaired hepatic or renal function • psychiatric patients • patients scheduled for elective surgery • pregnancy • women of childbearing age.

Dosage

Adult: Usual effective dose is 30 mg/d PO in divided doses. If no improvement is seen within 2 wk, increase dosage in 10 mg/d increments of 1–3 wk. May be increased to a maximum of 60 mg/d.

Pediatric Adolescent: Not recommended for children <16 y.

Geriatric: Patients >60 y are more prone to develop adverse effects; use with caution.

Dosage Forms: Tablets: 10 mg.

Pharmacokinetics

Absorption: rapidly from the GI tract. *Distribution:* crosses placenta and passes into breast milk. *Metabolism:* hepatic; $T_{1/2}$: unknown. *Elimination:* urine.

Adverse Effects

CV: Hypertensive crises, sometimes fatal, sometimes with intracranial bleeding, usually attributable to ingestion of contraindicated food or drink containing tyramine (see "Clinically Important Drug–Food Interactions" below); symptoms include some or all of the following: occipital headache that may radiate frontally; palpitations; neck stiffness or soreness; nausea; vomiting; sweating; dilated pupils; photophobia; tachy- or bradycardia; chest pain; orthostatic hypotension sometimes associated with falling; disturbed cardiac rate and rhythm, palpitations.

CNS: Dizziness, vertigo, headache, overactivity, hyperreflexia, tremors, muscle twitching, mania, hypomania, jitteriness, confusion, memory impairment, insomnia, weakness, fatigue, drowsiness, restlessness, overstimulation, increased anxiety, agitation, blurred vision, sweating, akathisia, ataxia, coma, euphoria, neuritis, repetitious babbling, chills, glaucoma, nystagmus.

GI: Constipation, diarrhea, nausea, abdominal pain, edema, dry mouth, anorexia, weight changes.

DERMATOLOGIC: Minor skin reactions, spider telangiectases, photosensitivity.

GU: Dysuria, incontinence, urinary retention, sexual disturbances.

OTHER: Hematologic changes, black tongue, hypernatremia.

Clinically Important Drug–Drug Interactions

⇇ Increased sympathomimetic effects (hypertensive crisis) when given with sympathomimetic drugs (norepinephrine, epinephrine, dopamine, dobutamine, levodopa, ephedrine), amphetamines, other anorexiants, local anesthetic solutions containing sympathomimetics.
⇇ Hypertensive crisis, coma, severe convulsions when given with tricyclic antidepressants (imipramine, desipramine etc.).
⇇ Additive hypoglycemic effect when given with insulin, oral sulfonylureas (tolbutamide, etc.).
⇇ Increased risk of adverse interactive actions if taken concurrently with meperidine.

Clinically Important Drug–Food Interactions

Tyramine (and other pressor amines) contained in foods are normally broken down by monoamine oxidase enzymes in the GI tract; in the presence of MAOIs, these vasopressors may be absorbed in high concentrations; in addition, tyramine releases accumulated norepinephrine from nerve terminals; thus, hypertensive crisis may occur when the following foods that contain tyramine or other vasopressors are ingested by a patient on an MAOI: dairy products (blue, Camembert, cheddar, mozzarella, Parmesan, Romano, Roquefort, Stilton cheeses; sour cream; yogurt); meats, fish (liver, pickled herring, fermented sausages—bologna, pepperoni, salami; caviar; dried fish; other fermented or spoiled meat or fish); beverages—undistilled (imported beer, ale; red wine—especially Chianti; sherry; coffee, tea, colas containing caffeine; chocolate drinks); fruit and vegetables (avocado, fava beans, figs, raisins, bananas, yeast extracts, soy sauce, chocolate).

Nursing Considerations

Assessment
• Assess for any conditions listed under "Contraindications/

Cautions" above.
• Assess for history or alcohol or drug dependence or abuse, use of currect prescribed or OTC drugs.
• Assess for suicidal ideation.
• Assess diet history for frequent use of any foods listed in "Clinically Important Drug–Food Interactions" above.
• Complete physical exam: vital signs, orthostatic BP, orientation, affect, reflexes, vision, liver and kidney function tests, urinalysis, CBC, ECG, EEG.
• Arrange for periodic liver function tests during therapy; arrange for discontinuation of drug at first sign of hepatic dysfunction or jaundice.
• Provide phentolamine or another alpha-adrenergic blocking drug on standby in case of hypertensive crisis.

Drug-Specific Patient Education
• Review the target symptoms that the drug potentially treats: depression.
• Review the dosing schedule until patient demonstrates a clear understanding of regimen.
• Review the most common side effects: dizziness, weakness or fainting when arising from a horizontal or sitting position; drowsiness, blurred vision; nausea, vomiting, loss of appetite; nightmares, confusion, inability to concentrate, emotional changes; changes in sexual function.
• Review the side effects patient should report promptly: headache, skin rash, darkening of the urine, pale stools, yellowing of the eyes or skin, fever, chills, sore throat, or any other unusual symptoms.
• Caution patient to avoid the ingestion of tyramine-containing foods or beverages while on this drug and for 10 d after drug is discontinued.
• Caution patient not to discontinue drug abruptly as serious side effects could occur.
• Caution patient to avoid the use of alcohol and sleep-inducing or OTC drugs.

TRAZODONE HYDROCHLORIDE

••••••••••••••••••••••••••

Desyrel

PREGNANCY CATEGORY C

Drug Classification: *Type:* proserotonergic antidepressant; *Class:* triazolopyridine derivative.

Mechanisms of Action

Presynaptic serotonin reuptake inhibitor; postsynaptic serotonin antagonism; adrenergic

receptor antagonism; norepinephrine reuptake inhibition.

Indications
Treatment of major depression;
anxiety symptoms associated
with depression; effective in
improving sleep duration
and quality; severe agitation
in geriatric patients.

Contraindications/Cautions
Contraindications: • hypersensitivity to trazodone
• pregnancy • lactation • EST
• recent MI • cardiac disease
• risk of toxicity and serotonin
syndrome with MAO inhibitor.
   Use cautiously with: • hepatic or renal impairment
• seizure history • may cause
hypomania or mania.

Dosage
Adult: 25–600 mg qd. May be
given qd or bid with major portion at hs. Consider trial a failure if patient shows no response on maximum
recommended dose after
4–6 wk.

Pediatric Adolescent: Safety and
efficacy not established for
children <18 y.

Geriatric: Give smallest adult
dose and increase slowly and
cautiously.

Dosage Forms: Tablets: 50, 100,
150, 300 mg.

Pharmacokinetics
Absorption: readily absorbed
from GI tract. *Distribution:*
crosses placenta; may enter
breast milk. *Metabolism:* hepatic; peak plasma level 2 h;
$T_{1/2}$: 6–11 h. *Elimination:* urine
and feces.

Adverse Effects
   CNS: Agitation,
nightmares/vivid dreams, hallucinations, delusions, hypomania, confusion, dizziness, incoordination, drowsiness, fatigue,
nervousness, blurred vision,
nasal/sinus congestion, malaise,
headache.
   CV: Hypertension, hypotension, shortness of breath, syncope, tachycardia, bradycardia,
palpitations.
   GI: Abdominal/gastric disorders, decreased/increased appetite, bad taste in mouth, dry
mouth, nausea, vomiting, diarrhea, flatulence, constipation.
   GU: Decreased libido and
sexual function, early menses,
missed periods, hematuria, delayed urine flow, increased urinary frequency; trazodone is
associated with the rare occur-
rence of priapism (approx.
1/7000 men) and permanent
damage to the penis may occur
without prompt medical or sur-
gical intervention.
   SKIN: Pruritus, rash.
   OTHER: Sweating, tinnitus,
weight gain/loss.

Clinically Important Drug–Drug Interactions

⫲ May increase digoxin or phenytoin levels.

⫲ Fluoxetine raises trazodone levels.

⫲ Increased depressant effects of CNS depressants.

⫲ Concurrent use with antihypertensives may cause hypotension.

Nursing Considerations

Assessment

• Assess for any of the conditions listed in "Contraindications/Cautions" above.

• Assess for concurrent prescription, OTC, or illegal drug or ETOH use/abuse; risk of suicide. Limit potentially suicidal patients' access to drug.

• Complete physical, vital signs, weight; CBC with differential; liver and thyroid function tests; BUN; creatinine; ECG if >40 y.

Drug-Specific Patient Education

• Review target symptoms that drug potentially treats: disruptions in sleep, appetite, concentration, energy, mood; anhedonia; interest; motivation; initiative; suicidal ideation.

• Review dosing schedule until patient demonstrates a clear understanding of regimen.

• Discuss expected lag period (3–4 wk) before full therapeutic effects can be anticipated.

• Review most common side effects (sedation, orthostatic hypotension, dizziness, nausea, headache) and encourage patient to report any side effects promptly.

• Educate patient about contraception during drug use.

• Caution patient about concurrent ETOH and drug use.

TRIFLUOPERAZINE HYDROCHLORIDE

Apo-Trifluoperazine (CAN), Stelazine

PREGNANCY CATEGORY C

Drug Classification: *Type:* dopamine receptor antagonist; also called antipsychotic, neuroleptic, or major tranquilizer; *Class:* phenothiazine; *Subclass:* piperazine.

Mechanisms of Action

Postsynaptic antagonism of dopamine receptors, primarily D2 (antipsychotic efficacy is thought to be mediated by these actions). Blockade of muscarinic cholinergic, noradrenergic, and histaminergic receptors (some undesirable side effects are thought to be mediated by these actions).

Indications

Short- and long-term management of idiopathic psychoses including schizophrenia, schizophreniform disorder, schizoaffective disorder, delusional disorder, brief psychotic disorder, mania with psychosis, and major depressive disorder with psychotic features.

Secondary psychoses associated with a general medical condition or substance-related disorder.

Acute deliria and organic psychoses.

Severe agitation or violent behavior.

Severe behavioral problems in children marked by combativeness and/or explosive hyperexcitability and in the short-term treatment of hyperactive children who show excessive motor activity.

Movement disorder of Huntington's disease.

Motor and vocal tics of Tourette's Syndrome.

Brief use for episodes of severe dyscontrol or apparent psychosis in some personality disorders.

Control of nausea, vomiting, and intractable hiccups.

Contraindications/Cautions

Contraindications: • allergy to trifluoperazine • comatose or severely depressed states
• presence of large amounts of CNS depressants (alcohol, barbiturates, narcotics, etc.)
• bone marrow depression
• blood dyscrasias • circulatory collapse • subcortical brain damage • Parkinson's disease
• liver damage • cerebral or coronary arteriosclerosis • CV disease • severe hypotension or hypertension • respiratory disorders • glaucoma • history of epilepsy or seizures • peptic ulcer or history of peptic ulcer
• decreased renal function
• urinary retention, ureteral or urethral spasm • prostate hypertrophy • breast cancer
• thyrotoxicosis • myelography within 24 h or scheduled within 48 h • pregnancy • lactation
• exposure to heat, rganophosphorous insecticides or atropine or related drugs • children with chickenpox • CNS infections • if signs and symptoms of tardive dyskinesia appear, drug discontinuation should be considered • history of Neuroleptic Malignant Syndrome.

Dosage

Adult: Patients may respond to widely different dosages of antipsychotics. Therefore, there is no set dosage for any given antipsychotic drug. Usual range for acute use (oral): 5–30 mg/d.

Usual range for maintenance use (oral): 5–75 mg/d. Can be administered once a day. IM: oral forms should be used whenever possible, but IM forms may be necessary for patients who exhibit violent behavior or for those who have high first-pass or presystemic metabolism of oral forms. Starting dose 2 mg IM; may repeat in 1 h; more than 6 mg/d is rarely needed. Switch to oral dosage as soon as patient is able or willing.

Pediatric Adolescent: Generally not used in children <6 y. Usual range 1–15 mg; IM 1–2 mg/d.

Geriatric: Start dosage at one-fourth to one-third that given in younger adults and increase more gradually.

Dosage Forms: Tablets: 1, 2, 5, 10 mg; Sustained release forms: 30, 75, 150, 200, 300 mg; Liquid concentrate: 10 mg/ml; Injection: 25 mg/ml; 2 mg/ml.

Pharmacokinetics

Absorption: (oral) adequate but variable; food or antacids may decrease absorption; liquid preparations are absorbed more rapidly and reliably than tablets; onset of action 3–60 min; peak level: 2–4 h; IM rapidly and reliably absorbed; onset of action 15–20 min; peak: 30–60 min. *Distribution:* highly protein bound (85–90%) and lipophilic; readily crosses the blood–brain barrier, placenta, and enters breast milk; concentrations in the brain appear to be greater than those in blood; not removed efficiently by dialysis. *Metabolism:* hepatic. *Elimination:* urine. The elimination half-life of most antipsychotic drugs is 18–40 h; plasma levels may vary among individuals by 10- to 20-fold.

Adverse Effects

CNS: Drowsiness, insomnia, vertigo, headache, weakness, tremors, ataxia, slurring of speech, cerebral edema, seizures, exacerbation of psychotic symptoms, extrapyramidal syndromes (EPS), neuroleptic malignant syndrome, tardive dyskinesia, pseudo-parkinsonism, akathisia (see descriptions of symptoms under "Implementation" below).

GI: Dry mouth, salivation, nausea, vomiting, anorexia, constipation, paralytic ileus.

CV: Hypotension, orthostatic hypotension, hypertension, tachycardia, bradycardia, cardiac arrest, CHF, cardiomegaly, refractory arrhythmias, dysrhythmias, pulmonary edema.

RESPIRATORY: Bronchospasm,

laryngospasm, dyspnea, suppression of cough reflex, and potential aspiration.

HEMATOLOGIC: Eosinophilia, leukopenia, leukocytosis, anemia, aplastic anemia, hemolytic anemia, thrombocytopenic or nonthrombocytopenic purpura, pancytopenia, elevated serum cholesterol.

GU: Urinary retention, polyuria, incontinence, priapism, ejaculation inhibition, male impotence, urine discolored pink to red-brown.

EENT: Nasal congestion, glaucoma, photophobia, blurred vision, miosis, mydriasis, deposits in the cornea and lens, pigmentary retinopathy.

HYPERSENSITIVITY: Jaundice, urticaria, angioneurotic edema, laryngeal edema, photosensitivity, eczema, asthma, anaphylactoid reactions, exfoliative dermatitis, contact dermatitis.

ENDOCRINE: Lactation, breast engorgement in females, galactorrhea, syndrome of inappropriate ADH secretion, amenorrhea, menstrual irregularities, gynecomastia, changes in libido, hyperglycemia, inhibition of ovulation, infertility, pseudopregnancy, reduced urinary levels of gonadotropins, estrogens, and progestins.

OTHER: Fever, heat stroke, pallor, flushed facies, sweating.

Clinically Important Drug–Drug Interactions

⊞ Additive anticholinergic effects and possibly decreased antipsychotic efficacy with anticholinergic drugs.

⊞ Additive CNS depression and hypotension with barbiturates, alcohol, meperidine.

⊞ Additive effects of both drugs with beta-blockers.

⊞ Increased risk of tachycardia, hypotension with epinephrine, norepinephrine.

⊞ Increased risk of seizure with metrizamide.

⊞ Decreased hypotension effect with guanethidine.

⊞ Because of displacement and competition for protein-binding sites, concomitant treatment with other highly protein-bound medications (e.g., warfarin, digoxin) could alter concentrations of both drugs.

⊞ Decreased effect of oral anticoagulants.

⊞ Possible increase in phenytoin levels.

Lab Test Interference

• False-positive pregnancy tests (less likely if serum test is used).

• Increase in protein-bound iodine not attributable to an increase in thyroxine.

• Blood levels of antipsychotics have not correlated well with clinical response and serum levels are probably more misleading than useful.

Nursing Considerations

Assessment

- Assess for any of the conditions listed under "Contraindications/Cautions" above.
- Assess for alcohol and drug use/abuse and for concomitant use of prescription and/or OTC medications.
- Assess for risk of suicidality.
- Complete physical exam: vital signs including orthostatic BP, ECG, CBC with differential, thyroid and liver function tests, BUN, creatinine.

Implementation

- Bioavailability differs between brand names of oral forms.
- Dilute liquid concentrate just before administration in 60 ml or more of fruit juice, milk, simple syrup, orange syrup, carbonated beverage, coffee, tea, water, or semisolid foods.
- Protect liquid concentrate from light.
- Give IM injection slowly into upper outer-quadrant of buttock.
- Be alert to potential for aspiration because of suppressed cough reflex.
- Monitor for dehydration, renal or liver abnormalities, depressed WBC, symptoms of infection. Promptly report to prescriber and institute remedial measures.
- Monitor for extrapyramidal side effects (involuntary dystonic muscular movements of the neck, jaw, tongue, or entire body; swallowing difficulties; oculogyric crisis); Parkinsonism (muscle stiffness; cogwheel rigidity; shuffling gait, stooped posture, drooling, coarse tremor, "rabbit syndrome," masklike facies, bradykinesia, akinesia); akathisia (subjective feeling of muscular discomfort that can cause agitation, restlessness, pacing, rocking, continually changing posture, and dysphoria).
- Monitor for symptoms of neuroleptic malignant syndrome: muscle rigidity; altered mental status; evidence of autonomic instability (e.g., irregular pulse or blood pressure, tachycardia, cardiac dysrhythmias); hyperpyrexia, sweating; increased WBC, blood creatinine phosphokinase, liver enzymes, myoglobin; mutism, obtundation, agitation.
- Monitor for symptoms of tardive dyskinesia (abnormal, involuntary, irregular, choreoathetoid movements of muscles of the head, limbs, and trunk; darting, twisting, and protruding movements of the tongue; chewing and lateral jaw movements; lip puckering; facial grimacing; finger movements and hand clenching; torticollis, retrocollis, trunk twisting,

pelvic thrusting).
• Taper drug gradually after high-dose therapy due to possible gastritis, nausea, dizziness, headache, tachycardia, insomnia after abrupt withdrawal.

Drug-Specific Patient Education
• Review target symptoms that drug potentially treats: auditory, visual, olfactory, tactile hallucinations; delusions; paranoia; disorders of thought and speech; psychotic agitation; insomnia.
• Review dosing schedule until patient demonstrates a clear understanding of regimen. Caution patient against changing dosage or discontinuation without consulting prescriber.
• Caution patient against concurrent alcohol or drug use.
• Discuss expected lag period (6 wk or more) before full therapeutic effects appear.
• Review most common side effects (drowsiness, insomnia, dry mouth, constipation, dizziness from hypotension, urinary hesitancy or retention, photosensitivity, blurred vision, urticaria, EPS, Parkinsonism, akathisia), and encourage patient to report any side effects promptly.
• If possible, give the patient full information about the risk of tardive dyskinesia and possible irreversibility. (The decision whether to inform patients and/or their guardians

must take into account the clinical circumstances and the competency of the patient to understand the information provided.)
• Educate patient about possibly life-threatening blood dyscrasias and instruct patient to report fever, chills, sore throat, unusual bleeding or bruising, or rash, and to discontinue medication immediately (most likely between 4th and 10th weeks of treatment).
• Caution patient about risk of dehydration or heat stroke, increased risk of sunburn, and warn against over exercising in a hot climate.

TRIFLUPROMAZINE HYDROCHLORIDE

••••••••••••••••••••••••••••

Vesprin

PREGNANCY CATEGORY C

Drug Classification: *Type:* antipsychotic, antiemetic, antianxiety; *Class:* dopaminergic blocking drug; *Subclass:* phenothiazine.

Mechanisms of Action
Blocks postsynaptic dopamine receptors in the brain; depresses those parts of the brain involved with wakefulness and emesis. Anticholinergic, antihistaminic (H1), and alpha-adrenergic blocking. Mecha-

nism of action not fully understood.

Indications

Management of manifestations of psychotic disorders, excluding psychotic depressive reactions.

Contraindications/Cautions

Contraindications: • allergy to triflupromazine • comatose or severely depressed states • bone marrow depression • circulatory collapse • subcortical brain damage.

Use cautiously with:
• Parkinson's disease • liver damage • cerebral or coronary arteriosclerosis • severe hypotension or hypertension • respiratory disorders • glaucoma • epilepsy or history of epilepsy • peptic ulcer or history of peptic ulcer • decreased renal function • prostate hypertrophy • breast cancer • thyrotoxicosis • myelography within 24 h or scheduled within 48 h • lactation • exposure to heat, phosphorous insecticides • children with chickenpox • CNS infections.

Dosage

Adult: 60 mg IM up to a maximum of 150 mg/d.

Pediatric Adolescent: >2 y: 0.2–0.25 mg/kg IM to a maximum of 10 mg/d.

Dosage Forms: Injection: 10, 20 mg/ml.

Pharmacokinetics

Absorption: rapidly from muscle. *Distribution:* highly protein-bound, widely distributed; crosses placenta and passes into breast milk. *Metabolism:* hepatic; $T_{1/2}$: 10–20 h. *Elimination:* urine.

Adverse Effects

CNS: Drowsiness, insomnia, vertigo, headache, weakness, tremors, ataxia, slurring, cerebral edema, seizures, exacerbation of psychotic symptoms, extrapyramidal syndromes; Neuroleptic Malignant Syndrome.

HEMATOLOGIC: Eosinophilia, leukopenia, leukocytosis, anemia, aplastic anemia, hemolytic anemia, thrombocytopenic or nonthrombocytopenic purpura, pancytopenia, elevated serum cholesterol.

CV: Hypotension, orthostatic hypotension, hypertension, tachycardia, bradycardia, cardiac arrest, CHF, cardiomegaly, refractory arrhythmias, pulmonary edema.

RESPIRATORY: Bronchospasm, laryngospasm, dyspnea, suppression of cough reflex and potential aspiration.

HYPERSENSITIVITY: Jaundice, urticaria, angioneurotic edema, laryngeal edema, photosensitivity, eczema, asthma, anaphylactoid reactions, exfoliative dermatitis, contact dermatitis with drug solutions.

ENDOCRINE: Lactation, breast engorgement in females, galactorrhea, syndrome of inappropriate ADH secretion, amenorrhea, menstrual irregularities, gynecomastia in males, changes in libido, hyperglycemia, inhibition of ovulation, infertility, pseudopregnancy, reduced urinary levels of gonadotropins, estrogens, and progestins.

GI: Dry mouth, salivation, nausea, vomiting, anorexia, constipation, paralytic ileus, incontinence.

EENT: Nasal congestion, glaucoma, photophobia, blurred vision, miosis, mydriasis, deposits in the cornea and lens, pigmentary retinopathy.

GU: Urinary retention, polyuria, incontinence, priapism, ejaculation inhibition, male impotence, urine discolored pink to red-brown.

OTHER: Fever, heatstroke, pallor, flushed facies, sweating, photosensitivity.

Clinically Important Drug–Drug Interactions

⸬ Additive anticholinergic effects and possibly decreased antipsychotic efficacy if taken concurrently with anticholinergic drugs.

⸬ Additive CNS depression, hypotension if given preoperatively with barbiturate anesthetics, alcohol, meperidine.

⸬ Additive effects of both drugs if concurrently with beta blockers.

⸬ Increased risk of tachycardia, hypotension if given concurrently with epinephrine, norepinephrine.

⸬ Increased risk of seizure if taken with metrizamide.

⸬ Decreased hypotension effect if taken concurrently with guanethidine

Nursing Considerations

Assessment

• Assess for any conditions listed under Contraindications/ Cautions" above.

• Assess for any history or alcohol or drug abuse or dependence, current use of prescribed or OTC medications.

• Assess for suicidal ideation.

• Complete physical exam: vital signs, orthostatic BP, intraocular pressure, ophthalmologic exam, CBC, urinalysis, EEG (as appropriate); thyroid, liver, and kidney function tests.

• Assure the injection is not given by SC injection; give slowly by deep IM injection into upper outer-quadrant of buttock.

• Assure that patient is kept recumbent for 30 min after injection to avoid orthostatic hypotension.

• Assess elderly patient for dehydration: sedation and decreased sensation of thirst owing to CNS effects can lead to dehydration, hemoconcentration, and reduced pulmonary ventilation; promptly institute remedial measures.

Drug-Specific Patient Education
• Review the target symptoms that the drug potentially treats: manifestations of psychoses.
• Review the dosing schedule until patient demonstrates a clear understanding of drug regimen.
• Review the most common side effects: drowsiness; sensitivity to the sun; pink or reddish-brown urine.
• Review the side effects patient should report promptly: sore throat, fever, unusual bleeding or bruising, rash, weakness, tremors, impaired vision, dark-colored urine, pale stools, yellowing of the skin and eyes.
• Caution patient to be careful in hot weather; may be prone to heatstroke while on this drug; encourage patient to keep up fluid intake and not exercise unduly in a hot climate.
• Caution patient to avoid sun exposure; use sunscreen and/or protective clothing.
• Caution patient not to stop

drug abruptly as serious side effects could occur.
• Caution patient to avoid alcohol and sleep-inducing or OTC mediations.

TRIHEXY-PHENIDYL HYDROCHLORIDE

• •

Apo-Trihex (CAN),Artane, Trihexy

PREGNANCY CATEGORY C

Drug Classification: *Type:* antiparkinsonian; *Class:* anticholinergic.

Mechanisms of Action
Has anticholinergic activity in the CNS that is believed to help normalize the hypothesized imbalance of cholinergic/dopaminergic neurotransmission created by the loss of dopaminergic neurons in the basal ganglia of the brains of Parkinsonism patients. Reduces severity of rigidity and also reduces, to a lesser extent, the akinesia and tremor that characterizes Parkinsonism. Less effective overall than levodopa. Peripheral anticholinergic effects suppress secondary symptoms of Parkinsonism such as drooling.

Indications

Adjunct in the treatment of Parkinsonism (postencephalitic, arteriosclerotic and idiopathic).

Adjuvant therapy with levodopa.

Control of drug-induced extrapyramidal disorders.

Contraindications/Cautions

Contraindications: • hypersensitivity to procyclidine • glaucoma, especially angle-closure glaucoma • pyloric or duodenal obstruction, stenosing peptic ulcers, achalasia (megaesophagus) • prostatic hypertrophy or bladder neck obstructions • myasthenia gravis • lactation. *Use cautiously with:* • tachycardia • cardiac arrhythmias • hypertension • hypotension • hepatic or renal dysfunction • alcoholism • chronic illness • people who work in hot environment • pregnancy.

Dosage

Adult: *Parkinsonism:* 1–2 mg PO the first day. Increase by 2 mg increments at 3–5-d intervals until a total of 6–10 mg is given daily. Postencephalitic patients may require 12–15 mg/d. Tolerated best if daily dose is divided into 3 (or 4) doses administered at mealtimes (and bedtime). *Concomitant use with levodopa:* Usual dose of each may need to be reduced; however, trihexyphenidyl has been shown to decrease bioavailability of levodopa. Adjust dosage on basis of response. 3–6 mg/d of trihexyphenidyl is usually adequate. *Concomitant use with other anticholinergics:* Gradually substitute trihexyphenidyl for all or part of the other anticholinergic and reduce dosage of the other anticholinergic gradually.

Drug-induced extrapyramidal symptoms: Initially 1 mg PO. If reactions are not controlled in a few hours, progressively increase subsequent doses until control is achieved. Dose of tranquilizer may need to be reduced temporarily to expedite control of extrapyramidal symptoms. Adjust dosage of both drugs subsequently to maintain ataractic effect without extrapyramidal reactions. *Sustained release preparations:* Do not use for initial therapy. Substitute on a mg for mg of total daily dose basis after patient is stabilized on conventional dosage forms. A single dose after breakfast or 2 divided doses 12 h apart may be given.

Pediatric Adolescent: Safety and efficacy not established.

Geriatric: Patients >60 often develop increased sensitivity to the CNS effects of anticholinergic drugs.

Dosage Forms: Tablets: 2, 5 mg; Sustained release capsules: 5 mg; Elixir: 2 mg/5 ml.

Pharmacokinetics

Absorption: rapidly from the GI tract. *Distribution:* widely distributed; crosses placenta and passes into breast milk. *Metabolism:* hepatic; T_{1_2}: 5.6–10.2 h. *Peak levels:* 1–1.3 h. *Elimination:* urine.

Adverse Effects
Peripheral Anticholinergic Effects

GI: Dry mouth, constipation, dilation of the colon, paralytic ileus.

CNS: Blurred vision, mydriasis, diplopia, increased intraocular tension, angle-closure glaucoma.

CV: Tachycardia, palpitations.

GU: Urinary retention, urinary hesitancy, dysuria, difficulty achieving or maintaining an erection.

GENERAL: Flushing, decreased sweating, elevated temperature.

CNS Effects, Some of Which Are Characteristic of Centrally Acting Anticholinergic Drugs

CNS: Disorientation, confusion, memory loss, hallucinations, psychoses, agitation, nervousness, delusions, delirium,

paranoia, euphoria, excitement, lightheadedness, dizziness, depression, drowsiness, weakness, giddiness, paresthesia, heaviness of the limbs, numbness of fingers.

OTHER: Muscular weakness, muscular cramping.

CV: Hypotension, orthostatic hypotension.

GI: Acute suppurative parotitis, nausea, vomiting, epigastric distress.

DERMATOLOGIC: Skin rash, urticaria, other dermatoses.

Clinically Important Drug–Drug Interactions

‡ Additive adverse CNS effects; toxic psychosis when given with phenothiazines.
‡ Possible masking of the development of persistent extrapyramidal symptoms, tardive dyskinesia, in patients on long-term therapy with antipsychotic drugs such as phenothiazines, haloperidol.
‡ Decreased therapeutic efficacy of antipsychotic drugs (phenothiazines, haloperidol).

Nursing Considerations
Assessment

• Assess for any conditions listed under "Contraindicaitons/ Cautions" above.
• Assess for history of alcohol or drug dependence or abuse,

use of current prescribed or OTC medications.

• Complete physical exam: vital signs, orthostatic BP, orientation, affect, reflexes, bilateral grip strength, visual exam including tonometry, liver and kidney function tests.

• Arrange to decrease dosage or discontinue drug temporarily if dry mouth is so severe that swallowing or speaking becomes difficult.

• Give with caution and arrange dosage reduction in hot weather as appropriate to patient's lifestyle; drug interferes with sweating and ability of body to maintain body heat equilibrium; anhidrosis and fatal hyperthermia have occurred.

Drug-Specific Patient Education

• Review the target symptoms that the drug potentially treats: drooling, lack of coordination, shuffling, speed impairment.

• Review the dosing schedule until patient demonstrates a clear understanding of regimen, including voiding before each dose if urinary retention is a problem.

• Review the most common side effect: drowsiness, dizziness, confusion, blurred vision; nausea; dry mouth; painful or difficult urination; constipation.

• Review the side effects patient should report promptly:

difficult or painful urination, constipation, rapid or pounding, heartbeat, confusion, eye pain, or rash.

• Caution patient to be careful in hot weather, the drug prohibits sweating increasing the susceptibility to heat prostration.

• Caution patient to avoid the use of alcohol and sleep-inducing or OTC drugs.

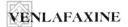

VENLAFAXINE

Effexor

PREGNANCY CATEGORY C

Drug Classification: *Type:* antidepressant; *Class:* phenylethylamine derivative.

Mechanisms of Action

Presynaptic reuptake inhibition of both serotonin and norepinephrine; not active at muscarinic, histaminergic, or alpha-one adrenergic receptors, or as an inhibitor of monoamine oxidase.

Indications

Treatment of depression; attention-deficit/hyperactivity disorder; pain syndromes.

Contraindications/Cautions

Contraindications: • hypersensitivity to venlafaxine

• pregnancy • lactation • hypertension • concomitant use with MAOIs.

Use cautiously with: • hepatic or renal impairment • seizure history • may cause hypomania or mania.

Dosage

Adult: 75–375 mg/d. Given bid or tid. Consider trial a failure if patient shows no response on maximum recommended dose after 4–6 wk.

Pediatric Adolescent: Safety and efficacy not established.

Geriatric: Start at 25 mg q a.m. and increase dose slowly and cautiously as tolerated.

Dosage Forms: Tablets: 25, 37.5, 50, 75, 100 mg.

Pharmacokinetics

Absorption: readily absorbed from GI tract. *Distribution:* not highly protein-bound; crosses placenta, may enter breast milk. *Metabolism:* hepatic; T_{1_2}: 5 h. *Steady state:* within 3 d. *Elimination:* urine.

Adverse Effects

CNS: Somnolence, insomnia, dizziness, nervousness, dry mouth, anxiety, tremor, asthenia, abnormal dreams, paresthesia, libido decreased, agitation, confusion, headache.

GI: Nausea, constipation, anorexia, diarrhea, vomiting, dyspepsia, flatulence.

CV: Vasodilatation, increased blood pressure/hypertension, tachycardia, postural hypotension.

SKIN: Sweating, rash, pruritus.

GU: Sexual dysfunction, urinary frequency, urination impaired, menstrual disorder.

OTHER: Blurred vision, yawning, taste perversion, tinnitus, mydriasis, weight loss.

Clinically Important Drug–Drug Interactions

⇥ Cimetidine may increase venlafaxine levels.
⇥ May increase depressant effects of CNS depressants.
⇥ Risk of toxicity and serotonin syndrome with MAOI.

Nursing Considerations

Assessment

• Assess for any of the conditions listed in "Contraindications/Cautions" above.
• Assess for concurrent prescription, OTC, or illegal drug or ETOH use/abuse; risk of suicide. Limit potentially suicidal patients' access to drug.
• Complete physical, vital signs, weight; CBC with differential; liver and thyroid function tests; BUN; creatinine; ECG if >40 y.

Drug-Specific Patient Education

• Review target symptoms that

drug potentially treats: disruptions in sleep, appetite, concentration, energy, mood; anhedonia; interest; motivation; initiative; suicidal ideation.

• Review dosing schedule until patient demonstrates a clear understanding of regimen.

• Discuss expected lag period (3–4 wk) before full therapeutic effects can be anticipated.

• Review most common side effects (sedation, sweating, dizziness, anorexia, nausea, vomiting, constipation, dry mouth, nervousness, tremor, asthenia, blurred vision, sexual dysfunction) and encourage patient to report any side effects promptly.

• Educate patient about contraception during drug use.

• Caution patient about concurrent ETOH and drug use.

ZOLPIDEM TARTRATE

• •

Ambien

PREGNANCY CATEGORY B

C-IV controlled substance

Drug Classification: *Type:* hypnotic; *Class:* imidazopyridine.

Mechanisms of Action
Modulates GABA receptors to cause suppression of neurons leading to sedation; has anti-convulsant, anxiolytic, and relaxant properties.

Indications
Short-term treatment of insomnia.

Contraindications/Cautions
Contraindications: • hypersensitivity to zolpidem.

Use cautiously with: • acute intermittent porphyria • impaired hepatic or renal function • addiction prone patients • pregnancy • lactation.

Dosage
Adult: Usual dosage is 10 mg PO at bedtime.

Pediatric Adolescent: Safety and efficacy not established.

Geriatric: Increased chance of confusion, acute brain syndrome; initiate treatment with 5 mg.

Dosage Forms: Tablets: 5, 10 mg.

Pharmacokinetics
Absorption: rapidly from the GI tract. *Distribution:* highly protein-bound; crosses placenta and may pass into breast milk. *Metabolism:* hepatic; $T_{1/2}$: 2.6 h. *Peak levels:* 1.6 h. *Elimination:* urine.

Adverse Effects
CNS: Convulsions, hallucinations, ataxia, EEG changes, pyrexia, morning drowsiness, hangover, headache, dizziness,

vertigo, acute brain syndrome and confusion; paradoxical excitation, anxiety, depression, nightmares, dreaming, diplopia, blurred vision, suppression of REM sleep; REM rebound when drug is discontinued.

GI: Esophagitis, vomiting, nausea, diarrhea, constipation.

HYPERSENSITIVITY: Generalized allergic reactions; pruritus, rash.

OTHER: Influenza-like symptoms, dry mouth, infection.

Nursing Considerations

Assessment

• Assess for any conditions listed under Contraindications/Cautions" above.

• Assess for history of alcohol or drug dependence or abuse, current use of prescribed or OTC medications.

• Assess for suicidal ideation.

• Complete physical exam: vital signs, orientation, affect, reflexes, vision exam, CBC with differential, hepatic and renal function tests.

Drug-Specific Patient Education

• Review the target symptoms that the drug potentially treats: insomnia.

• Review the dosing schedule until patient demonstrates clear understanding of regimen; note that long-term use is not recommended.

• Review the most common side effects: drowsiness, dizziness, blurred vision, GI upset.

• Review the side effects patient should report promptly: skin rash, sore throat, fever, bruising.

• Caution patient that drug must be withdrawn slowly after long-term use (not recommended) as serious side effects could occur.

• Caution patient to avoid alcohol, other sleep-inducing and OTC medications.

Index

The letter *t* following a number indicates tabular material; bold-face indicates major textual discussions.